CLINICAL DECISION MAKING

Case Studies in Maternity and Pediatric Nursing

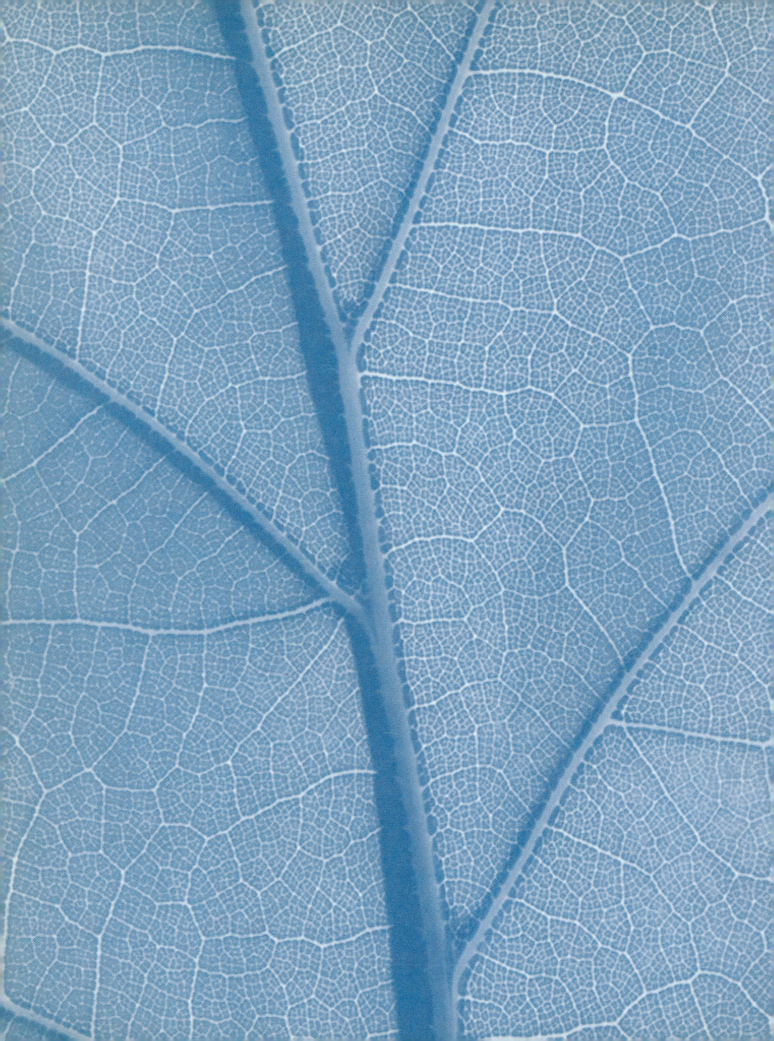

CLINICAL DECISION MAKING

Case Studies in Maternity and Pediatric Nursing

Diann S. Gregory
ARNP, CNM, MSEd

Professor of Nursing
MIAMI DADE COLLEGE, MIAMI, FLORIDA

Bonita Broyles
RN, BSN, MA, PhD

Instructor
ADN PROGRAM, PIEDMONT COMMUNITY COLLEGE,
NORTH CAROLINA

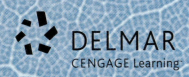

DELMAR
CENGAGE Learning

Australia   Canada   Mexico   Singapore   Spain   United Kingdom   United States

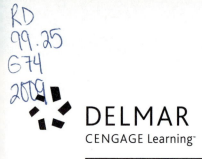

DELMAR
CENGAGE Learning™

**Clinical Decision Making: Case Studies
in Maternity and Pediatric Nursing**
Diann S. Gregory and Bonita Broyles

Vice President, Career and Professional
Editorial: Dave Garza

Director of Learning Solutions:
Matthew Kane

Acquisitions Editor: Maureen Rosener

Managing Editor: Marah Bellegarde

Product Manager: Patricia Gaworecki

Editorial Assistant: Meaghan O'Brien

Vice President, Career and Professional
Marketing: Jennifer McAvey

Marketing Director: Wendy Mapstone

Marketing Manager: Michele McTighe

Marketing Coordinator: Scott Chrysler

Production Director: Carolyn Miller

Production Manager: Andrew Crouth

Content Project Manager: Anne Sherman

Art Director: Jack Pendleton

Library of Congress Control Number: 2008930307

ISBN-13: 978-1-435-43983-2
ISBN-10: 1-4354-3983-X

Delmar Cengage Learning
5 Maxwell Drive
Clifton Park, NY 12065-2919
USA

Cengage Learning products are represented in Canada by Nelson Education, Ltd.

For your lifelong learning solutions, visit **delmar.cengage.com**

Visit our corporate website at **cengage.com**

Notice to the Reader
Publisher does not warrant or guarantee any of the products described herein or perform any
independent analysis in connection with any of the product information contained herein.
Publisher does not assume, and expressly disclaims, any obligation to obtain and include information other than that provided to it by the manufacturer. The reader is expressly warned to
consider and adopt all safety precautions that might be indicated by the activities described
herein and to avoid all potential hazards. By following the instructions contained herein, the
reader willingly assumes all risks in connection with such instructions. The publisher makes no
representations or warranties of any kind, including but not limited to, the warranties of fit-
ness for particular purpose or merchantability, nor are any such representations implied with
respect to the material set forth herein, and the publisher takes no responsibility with respect
to such material. The publisher shall not be liable for any special, consequential, or exemplary
damages resulting, in whole or part, from the readers' use of, or reliance upon, this material.

Printed in the United States of America
1 2 3 4 5 6 7 12 11 10 09 08

Contents

Section 1
Maternity Nursing

Comprehensive Table of Variables

CASE STUDY	AGE	SETTING	CULTURAL CONSIDERATIONS	ETHNICITY	PRE-EXISTING CONDITION	CO-EXISTING CONDITION/CURRENT PROBLEM	COMMUNICATIONS	DISABILITY	SOCIOECONOMIC STATUS	SPIRITUAL/RELIGIOUS	PSYCHOSOCIAL	LEGAL	ETHICAL	PRIORITIZATION	DELEGATION	PHARMACOLOGIC	ALTERNATIVE THERAPY	SIGNIFICANT HISTORY
Part 1: Prenatal Case Studies																		
1	23	Midwifery private practice		White American		×					×					×		×
2	17	Indian Reservation Clinic	Native American traditions	Native American						×	×					×		×
3	23	Certified Nurse Midwifery office	Recent Nigerian immigrant	African	×	×	×				×					×		×
4	36	Birth center	Rural American culture	White American	×	×				×			×					×
5	Adolescent	Prenatal clinic	Rastafarian Jamaican traditions	Jamaican	×	×										×		
6	43	Women's clinic	White middle-class American culture	White American	×	×												×
7	26	Prenatal clinic	Caribbean culture	Hispanic American	×	×	×		×	×	×	×	×	×		×		×
8	23	Private prenatal office	Mexican traditional health beliefs	Hispanic American	×	×								×		×	×	×
9	36	Free clinic		White American		×			×			×	×					
10	16	Prenatal clinic		White American				×						×				×
11	28	Birth center prenatal clinic	Native American traditions	Native American	×	×	×			×	×					×		×
Part 2: Intrapartum Case Studies																		
1	19	Certified Nurse Midwifery office/phone triage	Middle-class White American culture	White American	×				×								×	×
2	29	Home		White American	×	×	×				×							
3	15	Hospital urgent care center	Puerto Rican traditional beliefs	Hispanic American	×	×	×	×	×	×	×	×	×	×		×		×
4	23	Private OB practice/hospital	Traditional Colombian culture	Colombian				×										×
5	21	Freestanding birth center		White American	×	×								×				×
6	24	Birth center to hospital transfer	Black-Muslim traditions	Black American	×	×				×						×		×
7	36	Hospital labor and delivery unit		Indonesian American	×	×												×
8	41	Hospital labor and delivery unit		White American		×										×	×	×

#		Setting	Cultural Context	Ethnicity
9	26	Birth center	American urban professional culture	White American
10	17	Hospital labor and delivery unit	Black American	Black American
11		Hospital labor unit		Varied
12	22	Hospital labor and delivery unit	Accepts American medicalization concepts of pregnancy and birth	Black American

Part 3: Newborn Case Studies

#		Setting	Cultural Context	Ethnicity
1	24 hours	Hospital postpartum unit		White American
2	Newborn	Hospital delivery room		Black American
3	18 hours	Postpartum unit	Cuban American immigrant traditions	Cuban
4	6 hours	Small community hospital nursery		Black American
5	48 hours	Home		Black American
6	24 hours	Newborn nursery		White American
7	3 hours	Hospital		White American
8	2 hours	Hospital NB nursery		White American

Part 4: Postpartum Case Studies

#		Setting	Cultural Context	Ethnicity
1	29	Hospital postpartum unit	White American culture	White American
2	23	Home		White American
3	24	Home	Cuban traditions	Cuban American
4	14	Clinic		White American
5	26	Hospital postpartum unit	Pakistani traditions	Pakistani
6	24	Hospital postpartum unit	Jamaican Rastafarian culture	Black American

Part 5: Well Woman Case Studies

#		Setting	Cultural Context	Ethnicity
1	15	Certified Nurse Midwife's office		White American
2	28	Women's clinic		Black American
3	36	Well Woman clinic		Black American
4	31	Certified Nurse Midwife's office		Hispanic American
5	36	Infertility specialty center	Shinto health beliefs	Asian American
6	48	Well Woman private clinic	Black American professional culture	Black American
7	68	Well Woman clinic	Advanced age	White American

Section 2
Pediatrics

Comprehensive Table
of Variables

Case Study	Gender	Age	Setting	Ethnicity	Cultural Considerations	Preexisting Conditions	Coexisting Conditions	Significant History	Communication	Disability	Socioeconomic	Spiritual	Pharmacologic	Psychosocial	Legal	Ethical	Alternative Therapy	Prioritization	Delegation
Part One: The Digestive and Urinary Systems																			
1	F	4	Home/clinic	White American									×	×				×	×
2	M	neonate	Hospital	White American		×					×			×				×	
3	F	4 months	Clinic	White American					×		×			×	×			×	×
4	M	4	Hospital	Mexican American	Hispanic	×		×			×		×	×				×	×
5	M	18 months	Hospital	Black American			×							×				×	
6	M	2 days	Hospital	White American									×	×				×	×
7	M	6	Hospital	Black American		×								×				×	×
8	F	neonate	Hospital	Spanish American										×				×	
9	F	14	Home/clinic/hospital	White American							×		×	×		×		×	×
10	F	14	Hospital	White American										×				×	
Part Two: The Respiratory System																			
1	F	2 months	Hospital	White American		×								×				×	
2	M	6	Hospital	Black American									×	×				×	×
3	F	9 months	Hospital	White American		×					×			×				×	×
4	F	8	Hospital	White American		×				×			×	×				×	×
5	F	4	Hospital	White American		×	×		×				×	×				×	×
6	M	4	Hospital	White American			×				×			×	×		×	×	
7	F	10 months	Clinic	White American			×							×					
Part Three: The Cardiovascular System and the Blood																			
1	F	14	Hospital	Black American		×								×				×	×
2	M	8	Clinic/hospital	White American			×			×	×		×	×				×	
3	M	11 months	Hospital	White American			×						×	×				×	×
4	M	1 month	Hospital	White American							×			×				×	×
5	F	9	Hospital	Black American							×			×		×		×	×

Part Four: The Skeletal, Muscular, and Integumentary Systems

	Sex	Age	Setting	Ethnicity	Notes
1	F	5	Hospital	Asian American	
2	F	neonate	Hospital/clinic	White American	
3	M	13	Emergency department	White American	
4	F	11	Health care provider's office/hospital	White American	
5	M	14	Hospital	Russian	Recent Russian immigrant

Part Five: The Nervous and Endocrine Systems

	Sex	Age	Setting	Ethnicity	Notes
1	F	7	Health care provider's office	Spanish American	
2	M	9	School/hospital	White American	
3	F	13	Hospital	White American	
4	F	16	Psychiatric unit	White American	
5	M	10	Hospital	White American	

Part Six: The Lymphatic System

	Sex	Age	Setting	Ethnicity	Notes
1	M	20	Hospital/home	White American	
2	M	11	Hospital	Black American	
3	M	10	Home	White American	
4	F	4	Hospital	White American	
5	F	13	Hospital	Middle Eastern	Iraqi
6	F	11	Health care provider's office	Black American	

Part Seven: The Reproductive System

	Sex	Age	Setting	Ethnicity	Notes
1	F	3 weeks	Home	White American	
2	F	16	Prenatal clinic	White American	

Abbreviations Commonly Used in Maternity Nursing

ABR . . . . auditory brainstem response

AFI . . . . amniotic fluid index

AFP . . . . alpha fetoprotein

AGCUS. . . . . atypical glandular cells of undetermined significance

AMA . . . . advanced maternal age

AROM . . . . artificial rupture of membranes

ARNP . . . . advance registered nurse practitioner

ASCUS. . . . . atypical squamous cells of undetermined significance

BMI . . . . body mass index

BMR. basal metabolic rate

BP. . . . . blood pressure

BPD . . . . bronchopulmonary dysplasia

BPP. . . . . biophysical profile

BTBV . . . . beat to beat variability

BV . . . . bacterial vaginosis

CBC . . . . complete blood count

CNM. . . . . certified nurse midwife

CVAT . . . . costovertebral angle tenderness

CVS . . . . chorionic villus sampling

CPD . . . . cephalopelvic disproportion

CPM. . . . . certified professional midwife

DIC . . . . disseminated intravascular coagulopathy

DVT. . . . . deep vein thrombosis

EBL. estimated blood loss

EFW . . . . estimated fetal weight

EOAD. . . . . evoked otoacoustic emission test

FH . . . . fundal height

FHT. . . . . fetal heart tone

FM. . . . . fetal movement

fob. . . . . father of the baby

FSE. fetal scalp electrode

FSH . . . . follicle-stimulating hormone

FTP. . . . . failure to progress

GBS . . . . group B streptococcus

hCG . . . . human chorionic gonadotropin

H&H . . . . hematocrit and hemoglobin

H&P . . . . history and physical

HA. . . . . headache

HELLP . . . . hemolysis elevated liver enzymes and low platelets

HRT. . . . . hormone replacement therapy

HSIL . . . high-grade squamous intraepithelial lesions

I&O. . . . . intake and output

IDM . . . . infant of diabetic mother

IUGR . . . . intrauterine growth retardation

IUP. . . . . intrauterine pregnancy

IUPC. . . . . intrauterine pressure catheter

KVO. . . . . keep vein open

LLQ. . . . . left lower quadrant

LNMP. . . . . last normal menstrual period

LOA. . . . . left occiput anterior

LSB . . . . lower sternal border

LSIL . . . . low-grade squamous intraepithelial lesions

LTV. long-term variablility

MAS . . . . meconium aspiration syndrome

MMS. . . . . multiple marker screening

NEC . . . . necrotizing enterocolitis

NST . . . . non-stress test

NSVD. . . . . normal spontaneous vaginal delivery

OCP . . . . oral contraceptive pills

ONTD. . . . . open neural tube defects

PDA . . . . patent ductus arteriosis

PID . . . . pelvic inflammatory disease

PMI . . . . point of maximal impulse

PPV . . . . positive pressure ventilation

PPW . . . . pre-pregnancy weight

PPROM . . . . preterm premature rupture of membranes

PROM . . . . premature rupture of membranes

PTL . . . . preterm labor

RDS . . . . respiratory distress syndrome

R/O . . . . rule out

r/t . . . . related to

S , D . . . . size less than dates

SIDS . . . . sudden infant death syndrome

SIL . . . . squamous intraepithelial lesions

SROM . . . . spontaneous rupture of membranes

STI . . . . sexually transmitted infection (also known as STD—sexually transmitted disease)

T . . . . temperature

TENS . . . . transcutaneous electrical nerve stimulator

Toc . . . . test of cure

TOP . . . . termination of pregnancy

TPN . . . . total parenteral nutrition

TTN . . . . transient tachypnea of the newborn

URQ . . . . upper right quadrant

UTI . . . . urinary tract infection

VBAC . . . . vaginal birth after cesarean

VE . . . . vaginal exam

VS . . . . vital signs

wga . . . . weeks gestational age

wnl . . . . within normal limit

Reviewers

Jane H. Barnsteiner RN, PhD, FAAN
Professor of Pediatric Nursing
University of Pennsylvania School of Nursing
Philadelphia, Pennsylvania

Diana Jacobson MS, RN, CPNO
Faculty Associate
Arizona State University, College of Nursing
Tempe, Arizona

Denise G. Link, NPC, DNSc
Women's Health Care Nurse Practitioner
Clinical Associate Professor
Arizona State University
Tempe, Arizona

Tamella Livengood, APRN, BC, MSN, FNP
Nursing Faculty, Northwestern Michigan College
Traverse City, Michigan

Vicki Nees, RNC, MSN, APRN-BC
Associate Professor
Ivy Tech State College
Lafayette, Indiana

Nancy Oldenburg RN, MS, CPNP
Clinical Instructor
Northern Illinois University
DeKalb, Illinois

Deborah J. Persell MSN, RN, CPNP
Assistant Professor
Arkansas State University
Jonesboro, Arkansas

Patricia Posey-Goodwin, MSN, RN, EdD (c)
Assistant Professor
University of West Florida
Pensacola, Florida

JoAnne Solchany RN, ARNP, PhD, CS
Assistant Professor, Family & Child Nursing
University of Washington
Seattle, Washington

Preface

Delmar Cengage Learning's Case Studies Series was created to encourage nurses to bridge the gap between content knowledge and clinical application. The products within the series represent the most innovative and comprehensive approach to nursing case studies ever developed. Each title has been authored by experienced nurse educators and clinicians who understand the complexity of nursing practice as well as the challenges of teaching and learning. All of the cases are based on real-life clinical scenarios and demand thought and "action" from the nurse. Each case brings the user into the clinical setting, and invites him or her to utilize the nursing process while considering all of the variables that influence the client's condition and the care to be provided. Each case also represents a unique set of variables, to offer a breadth of learning experiences and to capture the reality of nursing practice. To gauge the progression of a user's knowledge and critical thinking ability, the cases have been categorized by difficulty level. Every section begins with basic cases and proceeds to more advanced scenarios, thereby presenting opportunities for learning and practice for both students and professionals.

All of the cases have undergone expert review to ensure that as many variables as possible are represented in a truly realistic manner and that each case reflects consistency with realities of modern nursing practice.

How to Use This Book

Every case begins with a table of variables that are encountered in practice, and that must be understood by the nurse in order to provide appropriate care to the client. Categories of variables include age; gender; setting; ethnicity; pre-existing conditions; coexisting conditions; cultural, communication considerations, disability, socioeconomic, spiritual, pharmacological, psychosocial, legal, ethical, prioritization, and delegation considerations; and alternative therapy. If a case involves a variable that is considered to have a significant impact on care, the specific variable is included in the table. This allows the user an "at a glance" view of the issues that will need to be considered to provide care to the client in the scenario. The table of variables is followed by a presentation of the case, including the history of the client, current condition, clinical setting, and professionals involved. A series of questions follows each case that ask the user to consider how she would handle the issues presented within the scenario. Suggested answers and rationales are provided for remediation and discussion.

Organization

The cases are grouped into parts based on topics. Within each part, cases are organized by difficulty level from easy, to moderate, to difficult. This classification is somewhat subjective, but they are based upon a developed standard. In general, difficulty level has been determined by the number of variables that impact the case and the complexity of the client's condition. Colored tabs are used to allow the user to distinguish the difficulty levels more easily. A comprehensive table of variables is also provided for reference, to allow the user to quickly select cases containing a particular variable of care.

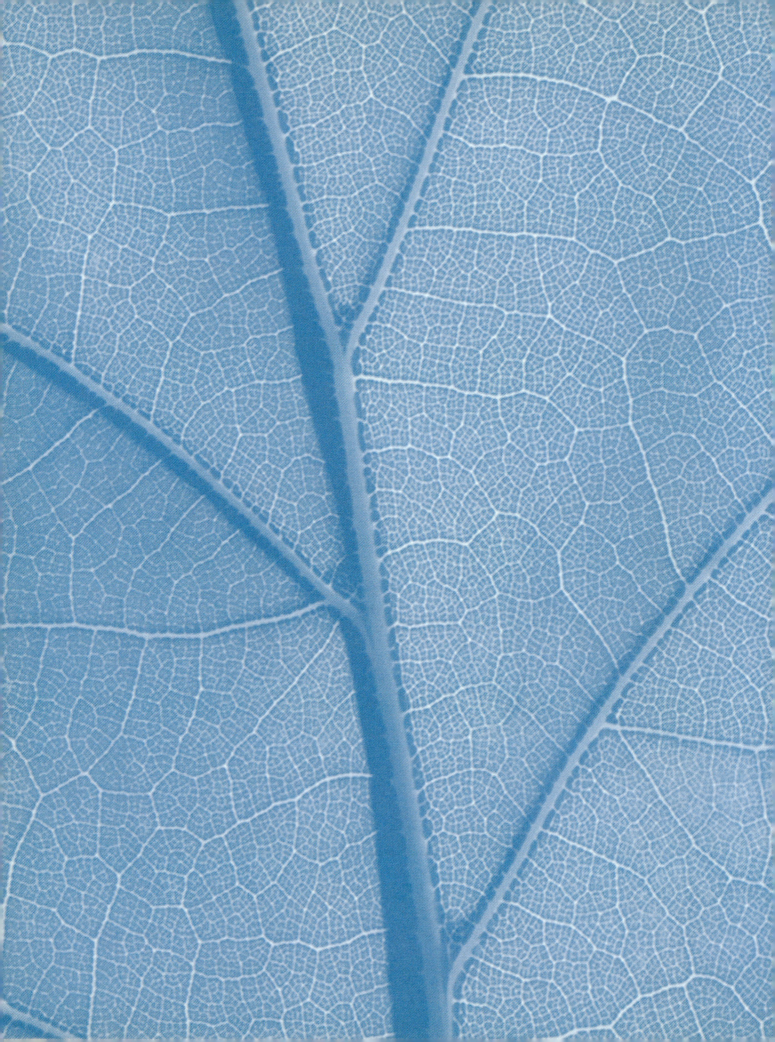

SECTION 1

CLINICAL DECISION MAKING

Case Studies in Maternity & Women's Health

Diann S. Gregory
ARNP, CNM, MSEd

Professor of Nursing
MIAMI DADE COLLEGE, MIAMI, FLORIDA

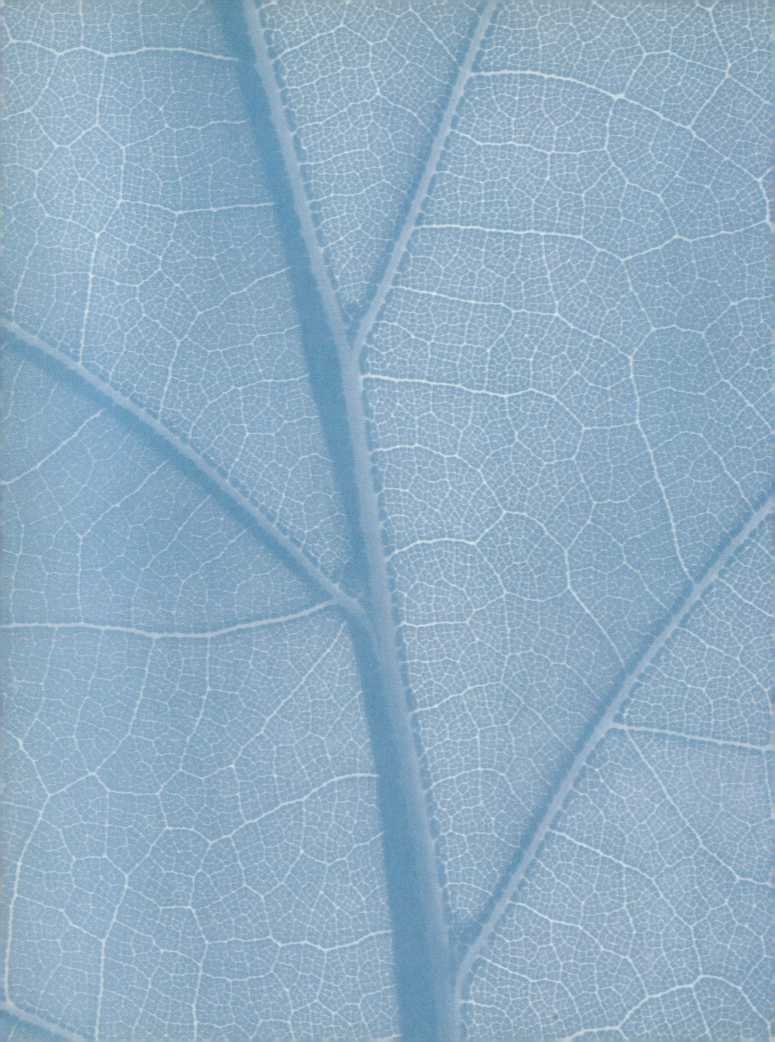

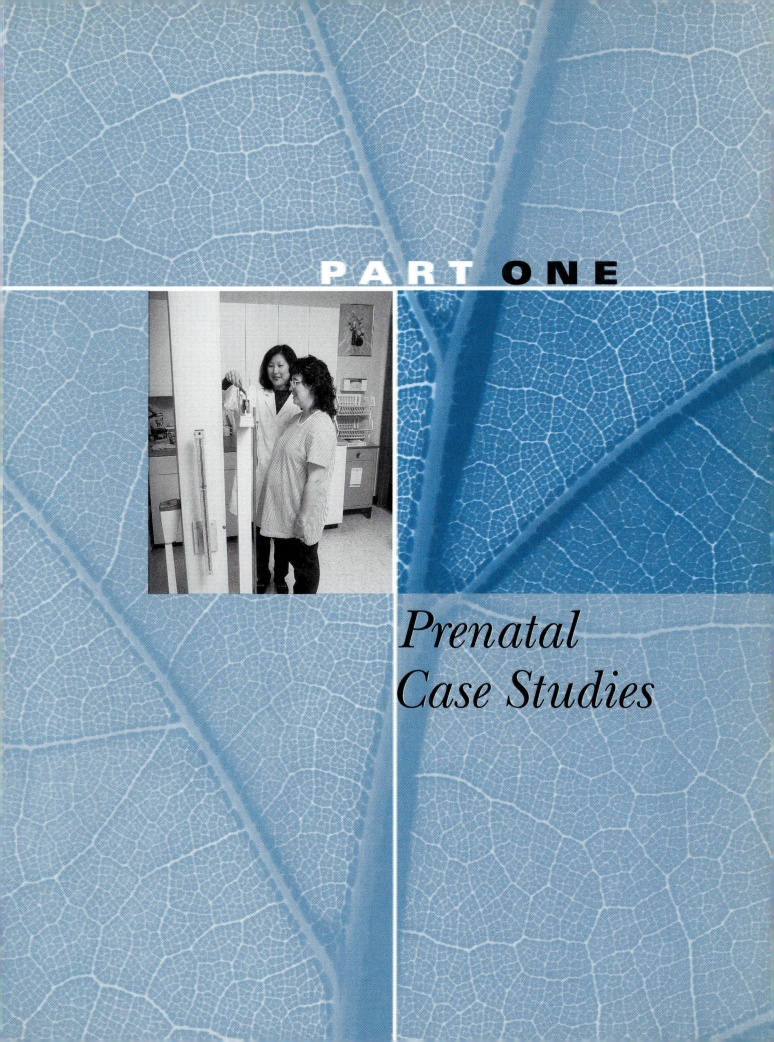

PART ONE

Prenatal
Case Studies

Linda

AGE

23

SETTING

■ Midwifery private practice

CULTURAL CONSIDERATIONS

ETHNICITY

■ White American

PRE-EXISTING CONDITION

CO-EXISTING CONDITION/CURRENT PROBLEM

■ Pregnant while taking oral contraceptives

COMMUNICATIONS

DISABILITY

SOCIOECONOMIC STATUS

SPIRITUAL/RELIGIOUS

PSYCHOSOCIAL

■ Trauma related to preterm birth/neonatal death

LEGAL

ETHICAL

PRIORITIZATION

DELEGATION

PHARMACOLOGIC

■ Metronidazole (Flagyl)
■ Oral contraceptives

ALTERNATIVE THERAPY

SIGNIFICANT HISTORY

■ Termination of pregnancy; preterm birth/neonatal death; multigravida

PRENATAL, second trimester

Level of difficulty: Easy

Overview: This case asks the student to respond to the mother regarding common changes that occur in pregnancy. It also asks the student to assess any risks associated with the mother using hormonal birth control during the early months of pregnancy.

Client Profile

Linda is a 23-year-old, married, White female (MWF). Linda went to see her family doctor after she had experienced two months of nausea and vomiting. She had been on birth control pills for two years and was certain that she could not be pregnant. The physician did a pregnancy test, and it was positive. Linda had often skipped periods when taking the pill and did not consider three months without a period unusual. She had been pregnant twice before. The first time was when she was 15 years old, and she had a first trimester elective abortion. The second time was three years ago, when she experienced a preterm birth at 28 weeks, and the baby died shortly after birth. That was a very traumatic experience for her, and she doesn't remember much about the pregnancy.

Case Study

Today is her first prenatal visit with her midwife. Linda's family doctor had sent her for an ultrasound and she brings the results with her to this appointment. It indicates that the pregnancy is at 14 weeks gestation. Her due date, or estimated date of delivery (EDD), is April 18. Linda has the following concerns: "I am worried about these bumps on my nipples, and why are my breasts so tender? Look at this line on my abdomen; where did that come from? I have this vaginal discharge. It doesn't itch or smell bad, but I notice I am a lot wetter than I have ever been before."

Questions

Respond to Linda's concerns:

1. "I am worried about these bumps on my nipples, and why are my breasts so tender?"

2. "Look at this line on my abdomen; where did that come from and what is the brownish coloring on my face?"

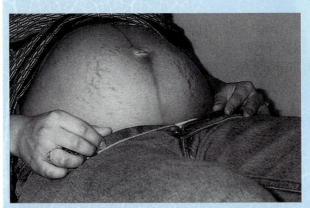

Figure 1.1 *Linea nigra.*

3. "Is it going to always be there?"

4. "I have this vaginal discharge. It doesn't itch or smell bad, but I notice I am a lot wetter than I have ever been before."

5. What is Linda's gravida/para?

6. Linda is very excited because her due date is on her birthday. She asks the nurse how certain it is that the baby will actually be born on that date. How should the nurse respond?

7. Linda admits that maybe she did miss a birth control pill several months ago. She continued to take them up to the day she saw her family doctor about the nausea and vomiting and found out she was pregnant. She asks the nurse how dangerous this might be to the baby she is carrying. How should the nurse reply?

8. Besides ultrasound, how can a due date be identified when there is no regular and accurate menstrual history to rely on?

9. Linda asks the nurse when she can first expect to feel her baby move. What is the best response by the nurse? What is this movement called?

10. Everything is normal at this initial visit. When should the nurse schedule Linda to return for her next prenatal visit?

11. Identify at least three areas of education that the nurse needs to address at this initial visit.

CASE STUDY 2

Aries

AGE	**SPIRITUAL/RELIGIOUS**
17	■ Native American traditions
SETTING	**PSYCHOSOCIAL**
■ Indian Reservation Clinic	■ No support from fob
CULTURAL CONSIDERATIONS	**LEGAL**
■ Native American traditions	
ETHNICITY	**ETHICAL**
■ Native American	
PRE-EXISTING CONDITION	**PRIORITIZATION**
CO-EXISTING CONDITION/CURRENT PROBLEM	**DELEGATION**
COMMUNICATIONS	**PHARMACOLOGIC**
	■ Fe supplementation
DISABILITY	**ALTERNATIVE THERAPY**
SOCIOECONOMIC STATUS	**SIGNIFICANT HISTORY**
■ Poverty	■ Primigravida

PRENATAL, second trimester

Level of difficulty: Easy

Overview: This case requires an understanding of Native American culture including the influence of the elders and taboos. It also reviews the risks associated with alcohol and tobacco in pregnancy.

Client Profile

Aries is a 17-year-old, single, Native American female, G1P0. She is five foot three inches tall and her pre-pregnant weight was 128 pounds. She is single and lives with her mother, two older sisters, and two older brothers in a small home near a reservation. Her father left the family when she was six months old. Her mother has managed to provide for the family by doing housekeeping for one of the wealthy families in town. They think the world of her mother and often give her bonuses to help with her financial problems. Aries and all of her siblings are embarrassed that their mother cleans houses and resent her employer's generosity. Her brothers, although 20 and 21 years old, cannot find work and just hang around the house or get into minor difficulties in town. One of her older sisters is in junior college studying to be a nurse, and the other is a senior in high school. Aries is the youngest and is a high school junior. Aries's grandmother lives nearby and often spends time at the house. It is Aries's grandmother who first brings her to the clinic for prenatal care.

Case Study

This is Aries's first prenatal visit. She had not been using any form of contraception. She did not intend to get pregnant, but did not take seriously the possibility that it could happen to her. Her last normal menstrual period was July 6 (today is November 20). When Aries is asked about her past medical history, the grandmother answers, but only vaguely. Aries is not able to tell the nurse how frequently her periods come. Aries is very respectful of her grandmother and sits quietly without making eye contact with the nurse during the interview. Aries does respond when asked about her use of alcohol and tobacco. She admits to drinking a little on weekends with her friends and smoking about 5 to 6 cigarettes a day. The baby's father boasts about the pregnancy but does not display any indication that he will assume any responsibility for the baby. Recently he has started dating another girl.

Questions

1. If Aries has a 28-day cycle, when is the baby due?

2. How many weeks gestation is she today?

3. What is the possible reason the nurse is having a problem getting a history from Aries and/or her grandmother regarding Aries?

4. What is the significance of Aries's grandmother bringing Aries to the initial prenatal visit?

5. How can the nurse obtain a better estimate of how much Aries drinks?

6. How much weight should Aries gain in the pregnancy?

7. List at least three risk factors associated with Aries's pregnancy.

8. Aries's grandmother instructs her to take herbs to improve her blood, but her sister (a nursing student) wants her to take iron supplements. Which advice do you think Aries will follow? Why?

9. Aries decides to quit school at 20 weeks gestation and stay close to home. She spends more time with her grandmother listening to stories while her grandmother works on quilts and macramé. They do not make anything for the baby. Why?

10. Aries is forbidden from working on the macramé. Why?

11. Give two common mistakes that nurses make when trying to provide care to women from cultures they are not familiar with.

CASE STUDY 3

Fayola

AGE

23

SETTING

- Certified Nurse Midwifery Office

CULTURAL CONSIDERATIONS

- Recent Nigerian immigrant

ETHNICITY

- African

PRE-EXISTING CONDITION

CO-EXISTING CONDITION/CURRENT PROBLEM

- Low back ache at 24 weeks gestational age (wga); r/o PTL; social isolation

COMMUNICATION

- Limited English

DISABILITY

SOCIOECONOMIC STATUS

SPIRITUAL/RELIGIOUS

PSYCHOSOCIAL

- Social isolation

LEGAL

ETHICAL

PRIORITIZATION

DELEGATION

PHARMACOLOGIC

- Tocolytics: ritodrine, terbutaline, magnesium sulfate, indomethacin, nifedipine nicardipine

ALTERNATIVE THERAPY

SIGNIFICANT HISTORY

- Primigravida

PRENATAL

Level of difficulty: Easy

Overview: Requires using critical thinking to identify those pieces of data that either rule in or rule out preterm labor.

Client Profile

Fayola is a 23-year-old G1P0 recent Nigerian immigrant. Her husband is an exchange student at the university doing graduate work in medicine. He works very long hours, leaving her alone most of the time. Her English is not good and she is very shy. She misses her family, especially now that she is pregnant. She started her prenatal care at 8 weeks gestation and looks to her midwife as a replacement mother. This has accounted for at least one phone call a week to the Certified Nurse Midwife (CNM) for one reason or another. Often these calls are just to receive reassurance.

Case Study

Fayola is now 24 wga. She calls the clinic to talk to her midwife with complaints of a low backache.

Questions

1. What are the most common reasons for backaches at 24 wga?

2. List at least five questions the nurse needs to ask Fayola about her backache to begin to assess the necessity of her coming to the clinic at this time.

3. What are Braxton Hicks contractions?

4. Is it common for women expecting their first babies to have uncomfortable Braxton Hicks contractions at this time in their pregnancies?

5. What are the typical characteristics of Braxton Hicks contractions?

6. What advice can the nurse give Fayola if she believes that the contractions are Braxton Hicks?

7. If the nurse suspects preterm labor, what should she advise Fayola to do?

8. Fayola goes to the hospital, where her contractions are timed at being 30 to 40 seconds and coming every 10 minutes. What further evaluation will be done to confirm if these are labor or Braxton Hicks contractions?

9. Fayola has not been drinking much for the past few days. How does dehydration relate to uterine contractions?

10. At the hospital triage Fayola's cervix was found to have no signs of preterm labor. She is given 500 ml of lactated Ringers IV solution, the contractions stop, and after two hours of observation, they discharge her with advice to drink more water on a regular basis. How much should she be drinking and how often?

11. Identify two nursing diagnoses that apply to Fayola at this time.

Lilly

AGE

36

SETTING

- Birth center

CULTURAL CONSIDERATIONS

- Rural American White culture

ETHNICITY

- White American

PRE-EXISTING CONDITION

- Breastfeeding a toddler while pregnant

CO-EXISTING CONDITION/CURRENT PROBLEM

- AMA; uncertain dates; infectious work environment; exposure to Fifth disease

COMMUNICATIONS

DISABILITY

SOCIOECONOMIC STATUS

SPIRITUAL/RELIGIOUS

PSYCHOSOCIAL

LEGAL

ETHICAL

PRIORITIZATION

- Breastfeeding; family dynamics

DELEGATION

PHARMACOLOGIC

ALTERNATIVE THERAPY

SIGNIFICANT HISTORY

- Multigravida

PRENATAL, second trimester

Level of difficulty: Moderate

Overview: Requires awareness of the risk associated with advanced age in pregnancy, exposure to teratogens, and family dynamics. The student is asked to assess effects of nursing a toddler while pregnant. Establishment of a due date with an unknown LNMP is also explored. This case also asks the student to consider factors that contribute to client satisfaction with the birth experience.

Client Profile

Lilly is a 36-year-old, G2P1001, MWF. Her last child, Katie, is 18 months old and is still nursing at night. Lilly is a certified day care worker in the toddler room at the local YWCA. She loves the job because it means she can be close to her daughter, who is in the room next door. Her husband owns his own landscaping business and enjoys working outdoors. Between them they make a comfortable living. They were just married three years ago and are pleased about this pregnancy since they want several children and feel that they got a late start. Their first daughter was delivered at the birth center. They were both very pleased with her birth and the care they received.

Case Study

Today is Lilly's first prenatal visit to the birth center with this pregnancy. Her husband and daughter accompany her. The nurse finds them in the waiting room going through the center's picture album. They find their picture from their daughter's birth and attempt to get Katie's interest. She briefly looks at it but is more interested in the toys in the children's corner. However, despite Katie's lack of interest, it is clear to the nurse that Lilly and her husband are enjoying reliving the experience through the pictures. After a brief discussion with Lilly and her husband, Lilly goes with the nurse to one of the exam rooms while her husband stays with Katie, who is busy with a set of blocks. The nurse begins Lilly's care by asking for information to establish her due date.

Questions

1. List three questions that the nurse may ask that will help establish Lilly's due date.

2. Lilly states that she first felt the baby move yesterday. If this is so, how far along might Lilly be?

3. As the pregnancy progresses, what other physical signs can be used to help confirm the due date?

4. Why is it important that Lilly's due date be determined during this early visit?

5. Identify two environmental risk factors that could possibly expose Lilly to teratogenic agents.

6. Identify at least two other risk factors for Lilly's pregnancy.

7. Lilly says that she is not ready to completely wean her 18-month-old from the breast. What advice should the nurse give her regarding this?

8. Lilly and her husband have decided that they want their daughter present for the labor and birth. What advice should the nurse offer them regarding this decision?

9. Lilly stated that one of the children at the child-care facility where she works has been diagnosed with Fifth disease. She asks if this is dangerous to her and her baby. How should the nurse respond?

10. What test will be done to determine if Lilly is at risk from Fifth disease?

11. Birth centers do not offer epidurals, and many do not offer any forms of medication for pain relief. Despite this, the level of satisfaction with birth center births is high, often higher than with medicated, hospital births. What factors affect how satisfied a woman is with her birth experience?

Florence

AGE

Adolescent

SETTING

- Prenatal clinic

CULTURAL CONSIDERATIONS

- Rastafarian Jamaican traditions

ETHNICITY

- Jamaican

PRE-EXISTING CONDITION

- Acne; possible teratogenic exposure; obesity; possible chronic hypertension

CO-EXISTING CONDITION/CURRENT PROBLEM

- Uncertain dating of pregnancy; hypertension

COMMUNICATIONS

DISABILITY

SOCIOECONOMIC STATUS

SPIRITUAL/RELIGIOUS

- Rastafarian

PSYCHOSOCIAL

- Much older male partner; denial of pregnancy; literacy; male dominant/female submissive behavior

LEGAL

- Minor (capacity to make decisions related to health care); privacy; state laws related to reporting statutory rape

ETHICAL

- Self-determination vs client advocacy

PRIORITIZATION

- Need to establish client age and due date; establishment of trusting relationship

DELEGATION

PHARMACOLOGIC

- Isotretinoin (Accutane)

ALTERNATIVE THERAPY

SIGNIFICANT HISTORY

PRENATAL

Level of difficulty: Moderate

Overview: Requires an awareness of adolescent behavior, Jamaican culture, and nonverbal communication. Requires awareness of prescription and OTC drug teratogenic potentials.

Client Profile

Florence, a Jamaican teen, presents at the prenatal clinic on August 20. As she registers at the reception desk the nurse begins her assessment by observing that an older male, who appears well groomed and in his late twenties or early thirties, accompanies her. The male companion is the one who fills out the registration information while Florence appears disinterested and casually leafs through a magazine. There doesn't seem to be any verbal exchange between Florence and her companion.

Florence is wearing an oversized sweatshirt and pants. Her hair is pulled back into a ponytail and she is wearing heavy foundation makeup, which may be meant to cover acne. She is wearing an opal pendant around her neck. She is approximately five feet three or four inches tall and the nurse estimates her weight at 160 pounds, although it is a little difficult to be certain with her baggy clothes. Florence continues to turn the pages in an almost automated manner without looking at the print or pictures.

Case Study

The nurse calls Florence's name in the waiting room to have her enter the intake room and begin her interview. As she stands up to follow the nurse, her companion also stands and begins to follow her. Florence seems to expect this. The nurse stops and explains that initially she always interviews new clients alone, but she respects his desire to be involved and will call him in later. At first both Florence and her companion are taken aback by this arrangement; however, the nurse's matter-of-fact approach and her warm manner and willingness to involve him "as soon as possible" put them both off guard and Florence follows the nurse alone.

The following additional data is collected:

FH 26 cm

Urine dip indicated negative protein, glucose; positive ketones, nitrites, and leukocytes

BP 138/84

Actual weight is 168 pounds (She states that her prepregnant weight was around 158 to 160 pounds.)

An ultrasound is done and it is determined that Florence is approximately 26 weeks gestation at this initial visit.

Questions

1. Discuss the significance of Florence's appearance and behavior.

2. Discuss the significance of the companion's behaviors.

3. Which of the following do you believe was the rationale for the nurse's behavior?

  a. She was establishing her authority in the clinic setting.

  b. She was protecting Florence's privacy during the health interview.

  c. She was letting the "man" know that, although he wishes to be involved, there will be a time and a place for his involvement.

  d. She desired to hear how Florence would answer questions, not how her companion would answer them for her.

4. During the interview Florence states that her last menstrual period was March 16. What is Florence's due date?

5. What questions need to be answered to determine how accurate this due date is?

6. What are the implications of her coming so late for prenatal care?

7. Nutrition is always important during pregnancy. State two reasons the nurse needs to be especially concerned about this client's nutritional habits.

8. Florence is covering her acne with a heavy makeup foundation. Some acne medications are known to be teratogenic. Which ones are dangerous, and when are they the most dangerous? What advice can the nurse give Florence regarding treatment for her acne during pregnancy?

9. What is the significance of the positive ketones in her urine?

10. What is the implication of the positive nitrites and leukocytes esterase in the urine?

11. Florence tells the nurse that her usual blood pressure is 118–120/65–75. Describe the normal blood pressure changes in pregnancy. Does Florence's blood pressure at this initial visit fit into the normal pattern expected for this time in her pregnancy?

Ruby

AGE

43

SETTING

■ Women's clinic

CULTURAL CONSIDERATIONS

■ White middle-class American culture

ETHNICITY

■ White American

PRE-EXISTING CONDITION

■ Obesity

CO-EXISTING CONDITION/CURRENT PROBLEM

■ AMA; perimenopausal; 2nd trimester spotting; high fundal height; hepatitis B vaccine; severe N&V

COMMUNICATIONS

DISABILITY

SOCIOECONOMIC STATUS

SPIRITUAL/RELIGIOUS

PSYCHOSOCIAL

LEGAL

ETHICAL

PRIORITIZATION

DELEGATION

PHARMACOLOGIC

ALTERNATIVE THERAPY

SIGNIFICANT HISTORY

■ Multigravida

MODERATE

ANTEPARTUM

Level of difficulty: Moderate

Overview: In the case the student is asked to assess perimenopausal symptoms and an unplanned AMA pregnancy as well as explores causes of early pregnancy spotting. This case also looks at vaccination during pregnancy.

Client Profile

Ruby is a 43-year-old, G4P2103, divorced White American female. Her youngest child is now 23 years old. Ruby is an art teacher at a local junior high school. She has been having unusually heavy, irregular periods for approximately six months, and then no period for the past three months. During these three months she has been very fatigued and experiencing nausea and vomiting twice a day. Ruby is five feet four inches tall, and her current weight is 140 pounds. Despite the nausea and vomiting, she has gained five pounds in the past three months.

Case Study

Ruby came to the women's clinic today to get information on menopause and to find out why she has been feeling so sick. A pregnancy test came back positive. Her physical exam confirmed a uterus enlarged to a 16 weeks size and FHTs were heard. Ruby is spotting. She just finished a series of injections of the hepatitis B vaccine. Ruby is in mild disbelief!

Questions

1. What is the most probable cause of her heavy irregular periods in the years just prior to the menopause?

2. What are the risks associated with this pregnancy?

3. What screening tests are available to screen for congenital anomalies?

4. What is Ruby's BMI? How much weight should Ruby gain?

5. List at least five common signs and symptoms of menopause.

6. When can a woman consider herself in menopause and therefore discontinue birth control?

7. What information can the nurse use to try to determine Ruby's due date?

8. Give four possible reasons for Ruby's spotting.

9. Ruby's fundal height is high for the dates she reports. Name two possible reasons for this, and explain your answers.

10. Are there risks associated with hepatitis B vaccine during pregnancy?

Caridad

AGE

26

SETTING

- Prenatal clinic

CULTURAL CONSIDERATIONS

- Caribbean culture

ETHNICITY

- Hispanic American

PRE-EXISTING CONDITION

CO-EXISTING CONDITION/CURRENT PROBLEM

- No fetal movement in 24 hours; fetal demise; tobacco use

COMMUNICATIONS

DISABILITY

SOCIOECONOMIC STATUS

SPIRITUAL/RELIGIOUS

PSYCHOSOCIAL

LEGAL

ETHICAL

PRIORITIZATION

DELEGATION

PHARMACOLOGIC

- Oxytocin (Pitocin)

ALTERNATIVE THERAPY

SIGNIFICANT HISTORY

- Primigravida

PRENATAL/INTRAPARTUM

Level of difficulty: Moderate

Overview: Requires using critical thinking to assess and care for a woman who has experienced an intrauterine fetal loss.

Client Profile

Caridad is a 26-year-old, G1P0, MHF at 28 wga. Her pregnancy thus far has been uneventful except for some spotting during the first six weeks. Caridad smokes 3 to 4 cigarettes a day.

Case Study

Caridad calls the prenatal clinic to say that earlier this morning she had felt her baby move a lot. She said the movement was so violent that it actually hurt her. Now she realizes that she has not felt her baby move again all day. She is told to come in, and the baby's heart tones are checked. They cannot be located. An ultrasound is ordered, and the diagnosis of fetal demise is made.

Questions

1. Is there a relationship between the spotting during the first trimester and later intrauterine fetal death (IUFD)?

2. Caridad is not experiencing any bleeding or cramping at this time. What is the probability that she will go into spontaneous labor soon?

3. If she does not go into labor, how will the pregnancy be terminated?

4. What are the risks for Caridad if she decides to wait for her body to naturally go into labor?

5. What lab work should the nurse anticipate for Caridad?

6. What emotional and/or psychological responses should the nurse anticipate from Caridad during her labor?

7. How might this experience affect Caridad in future pregnancies?

8. How might the nurse guide Caridad's family to support her during this time?

9. How likely is it that her smoking caused the fatal demise?

10. After two weeks it is determined that Caridad needs to be induced. Her cervix is still long and closed, firm and midline. Describe how prostaglandins can be used to prepare the cervix for induction. Include nursing responsibilities related to safety during this procedure.

C A S E   S T U D Y   8

Esparanza

AGE

23

SETTING

- Private prenatal office

CULTURAL CONSIDERATIONS

- Mexican traditional health beliefs

ETHNICITY

- Hispanic American

PRE-EXISTING CONDITION

- Previous breech birth

CO-EXISTING CONDITION/CURRENT PROBLEM

- Breech presentation

COMMUNICATIONS

DISABILITY

SOCIOECONOMIC STATUS

SPIRITUAL/RELIGIOUS

PSYCHOSOCIAL

LEGAL

ETHICAL

- Client needs vs practitioner's needs

PRIORITIZATION

- Safety vs client desire for VBAC

DELEGATION

PHARMACOLOGIC

- RhoGAM

ALTERNATIVE THERAPY

- Moxibustion; light; music

SIGNIFICANT HISTORY

- Multigravida; previous cesarean section

PRENATAL

Level of difficulty: Difficult

Overview: Requires knowledge regarding breech presentations and cesarean section. This case asks students to use critical thinking to compare and contrast VBAC and cesarean section and the types of anesthesia used.

Client Profile

Esparanza is a 23-year-old, G2P1001, MHF at 36 wga. She had a previous cesarean section with an epidural in Mexico six years ago for a breech presentation at 38 weeks gestational age. The baby weighed six pounds. She is five feet two inches tall, and her PPW was 100 pounds. She would like a vaginal birth after cesarean section (VBAC) with this pregnancy, however she saw six doctors before she found one who would even consider doing a VBAC.

Case Study

Esparanza seems anxious at today's prenatal visit. She tells the nurse that the baby feels like his head is up under her ribs and she fears another cesarean section for breech. The following data is obtained at this visit:

    Wt 125 lb

    FHT 140s URQ

    Fundal height (FH) 35 cm

    Fetal movement +(FM)

    Urine chemstrip testing: all negative

    No HA, vision changes

    No CVAT

    No edema

Questions

1. Why was it so difficult for Esparanza to find an obstetrician who would consider doing a VBAC? Discuss the ethical dilemmas that exist when the desires and needs of the client come in conflict with those of the practitioner.

2. What are the routine labs for this visit, and why are they done at this time?

3. Compare and contrast VBAC and repeat cesarean section for the following: safety for both mother and baby, cost, pain; long-term effects, effects on breastfeeding, and parenting.

4. Her obstetrician asks for her previous cesarean section records before he will even consider a VBAC. Why?

5. Why are cesarean sections usually done for breech presentation?

6. When would a vaginal delivery be considered for a breech presentation?

7. How can the baby be encouraged to move to a cephalic presentation?

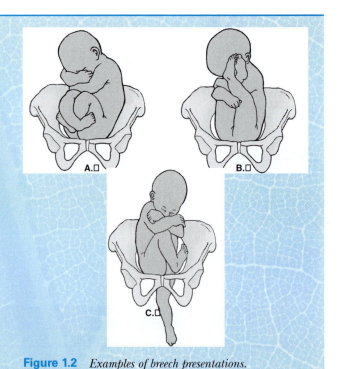

Figure 1.2 *Examples of breech presentations.*

8. What maternal/fetal conditions contribute to a baby presenting in a breech presentation?

9. Compare and contrast spinal and epidural anesthesia for cesarean section.

10. If the baby changes to a cephalic presentation in the next two weeks but Esparanza does not go into spontaneous labor, can she be safely induced for a VBAC?

11. What methods can be used if any?

12. Esparanza begins to cry at the 39-week visit when she realizes that the baby has not yet changed position. She says that "I just know it's going to be terrible again. I'll never be able to breastfeed my baby postpartum; it's so painful." How should the nurse respond?

Sarah

AGE

36

SETTING

- Free clinic

CULTURAL CONSIDERATIONS

ETHNICITY

- White American

PRE-EXISTING CONDITION

CO-EXISTING CONDITION/CURRENT PROBLEM

- Uncertain EDC; financial problems; yeast infection

COMMUNICATIONS

DISABILITY

SOCIOECONOMIC STATUS

- Low income (no health insurance)

SPIRITUAL/RELIGIOUS

PSYCHOSOCIAL

LEGAL

ETHICAL

- Need for care vs ability to pay

PRIORITIZATION

DELEGATION

PHARMACOLOGIC

ALTERNATIVE THERAPY

SIGNIFICANT HISTORY

- Adopted; history of pregnancy loss— 2 spontaneous abortions, 1 preterm loss; mulitgravida

PRENATAL

Level of difficulty: Difficult

Overview: Requires identification of history strongly suggestive of diabetes. Requires critical thinking to set priorities for care. Ask students to consider social responsibility concerns.

DIFFICULT

Client Profile

Sarah is a 36-year-old, G4P0120, MWF at approximately 18 weeks gestation at her initial PNV (according to unsure dates and uterine size). She presents to a reduced fee clinic run by the Kiwanis Club. She is five feet three inches and her pre-pregnant weight was 136 pounds.

Case Study

Her chief complaints at this visit include positive pregnancy test five weeks ago, vaginal discharge (white cheesy odorless), and pruritus. Her medical history includes recurrent urinary tract infections and yeast infections. She has a negative surgical history. She was adopted and does not know her family history. Significant OB history includes two spontaneous abortions (SAB). One was three years ago at 12 weeks and one was six months ago at 10 to 12 weeks. She also had a loss of a 32-week infant following complications associated with preterm premature rupture of membranes (PPROM) two years ago. The infant weighed 8 pounds and died from respiratory distress syndrome (RDS) and sepsis (early onset GBS). The baby lived 14 hours and also experienced jaundice, hypoglycemia, temperature instability, and acidosis.

Sarah and her husband both work two part-time jobs each. They have no health insurance and earn too much for Medicaid. Although they manage to pay their bills, there is seldom anything left for health care. Subsequently, neither one is able to receive regular checkups. As a matter of fact, the last time Sarah saw a doctor was when she went into labor with her preterm baby two years ago. (She was not receiving prenatal care for that pregnancy.) When she had her last SAB she bled for about two months but did not seek medical care. She felt that she had been through this before and that it would stop on its own. It did, and she resumed work after several weeks. They are still paying for her last hospitalization and the bills for the baby they lost. This accounts for why she waited until 18 weeks to seek prenatal care at this time. She might have waited longer except that a friend told her about the Kiwanis clinic and suggested that she might be able to afford care there.

Today she tells you that, although they have the money for the $20 office visit, they only have enough money to pay for some of the lab work. This couple does not want to return to the county hospital because they do not qualify for any financial relief, and the cost of care for those who have to pay at the county hospital is very high. The only advantages the county hospital holds for them are that they can receive care (will not be turned away) and they can make small payments. They already feel that they will spend the rest of their lives trying to pay off the preterm baby they lost, and they do not wish to add to their debt for this pregnancy. Like many couples they "slip through the cracks" in our medical system and have little choice for care. They ask the nurse what lab tests they *really need* to have done at this time and which ones can wait until they can bring in more money.

Questions

1. Based on Sarah's obstetrical history, list two major concerns for this pregnancy.

2. Review what is included in initial prenatal lab work. She is already approximately 18 weeks. What lab work is crucial for her at this time, and what can safely wait?

3. What other sources might you direct this couple to for financial help?

4. Can you predict any prenatal complications from the data previously given?

5. If this couple lived in your hometown, what would be the options open to them for care?

6. Discuss the following statement: "Not providing adequate prenatal care is much more expensive than providing it."

7. If you were in a political position to change the health care system regarding maternity care, how would you change it?

8. As a student, what can you do to bring situations like this to the forefront so that individuals who have the power to change things will respond?

9. Discuss your professional responsibility to become involved in policy decision making regarding availability of medical care.

10. Free clinics (those that only charge the exact cost of supplies used) or reduced-cost clinics are sometimes able to provide care at much lower fees than mainstream care facilities. Sometimes free clinics are subsidized to be able to provide care at no cost. One reason they can do that is volunteer professional help. In the past, charitable facilities were protected from lawsuits by sovereign immunity. This protection has been removed in many areas. What is the status in your area? How does having, or not having, sovereign immunity affect the cost of health care? Discuss the pros and cons of these legal changes.

Kathie

AGE

16

SETTING

- Prenatal clinic

CULTURAL CONSIDERATIONS

ETHNICITY

- White American

PRE-EXISTING CONDITION

CO-EXISTING CONDITION/CURRENT PROBLEM

- UTI/kidney; BV; HPV; severe N&V with weight loss; uncertain due date

COMMUNICATIONS

- Third-grade reading level

DISABILITY

SOCIOECONOMIC STATUS

- Lives with grandmother in subsidized housing; poverty

SPIRITUAL/RELIGIOUS

PSYCHOSOCIAL

- Third-grade educational level; unrealistic expectations; fob is married

LEGAL

- Statutory rape

ETHICAL

PRIORITIZATION

- Need to establish client age and due date; establishment of trusting relationship

DELEGATION

PHARMACOLOGIC

ALTERNATIVE THERAPY

SIGNIFICANT HISTORY

- Primigravida

DIFFICULT

PRENATAL

Level of difficulty: Difficult

Overview: Requires that the nurse understand some of the misconceptions common among teens with low literacy levels regarding their sexuality, fantasy thinking, and health problems often related to these misconceptions and unsafe behaviors.

Client Profile

Kathie is a 16-year-old, SWF who has missed four periods. She lives with her grandmother. The grandmother raised her and her two sisters. Kathie is the youngest. One of her sisters has two children. They all live together in a three-bedroom, subsidized apartment. Kathie is five feet six inches, and her current weight is 110 lbs. As far as she can remember, her pre-pregnant weight was 108. She states that the fob, a 28-year-old married man, denies this is his baby. Kathie states that she is not worried, that he will "come around and love this baby." Kathie attends an overcrowded, inner-city high school and is a junior. She can neither read nor write above the third-grade level. She tells the midwife that when she graduates she wants to become a doctor.

Case Study

Kathie can't believe that she is pregnant since she had been douching for birth control every time she had intercourse. She complains of excessive vomiting and states that she has lost 10 pounds in the past two weeks. Other complaints include intermittent chills, pain in the lower right back area, and pain with voiding. She has dark circles under her eyes and her mucus membranes are dry and pale. Her vital signs are: BP 108/68, T 103.8°F, P 88, and R 22.

Upon examining the midwife notes:

1. Right side, cervical lymph glands are enlarged and tender
2. Needs dental work on two of her upper right molars
3. Fundal height is three fingers below the umbilicus
4. FHT are heard in the LLQ (130s)
5. When doing her PAP the midwife notes that she has a homogenous gray clinging discharge with a pH of 5.5
6. The wet mount has clue cells (epithelial cells with a stippled appearance)
7. The whiff test (a fishy odor when potassium hydroxide is added to the vaginal secretions) is also positive
8. Wart-like growths on the outside of her vagina with positive ascetic-white test
9. Urine chemstrip in the office is positive for ketones, nitrites, and leukocytes; negative for glucose and protein.

Kathie is given HIV counseling and agrees to be tested. Her HIV test comes back negative.

Questions

1. If Kathie's size equals her dates, about how many weeks pregnant do you think she is?

2. Why do you think she put off coming in for prenatal care so long?

3. How important is it that her due date be established at this first visit?

4. In light of Kathie's advanced gestation and weight loss, how significant is her nausea and vomiting?

5. Which of Kathie's signs and symptoms point to a urinary tract infection? How serious are these signs and symptoms?

6. What are the implications of UTI for pregnancy?

7. What is the significance of the homogenous gray clinging discharge, positive whiff test, and finding of the clue cells?

8. What are vaginal warts that turn white with ascetic acid probably caused by?

9. What is the most likely reason Kathie has swollen cervical lymph glands?

10. What are the implications of dental caries/infections for pregnancy?

11. Discuss common misconceptions teens have about contraception.

12. Make a list of topics the nurse should discuss with Kathie as a result of the initial exam.

13. Make a list of topics to be discussed with Kathie regarding a healthy pregnancy.

14. In light of Kathie's reading level, how will the nurse provide education?

Ruth

AGE

28

SETTING

- Birth center prenatal clinic

CULTURAL CONSIDERATIONS

- Native American traditions

ETHNICITY

- Native American

PRE-EXISTING CONDITION

- Asthma; obesity

CO-EXISTING CONDITION/CURRENT PROBLEM

- Late entry into care; multiple gestation; blurred vision; tobacco use

COMMUNICATIONS

DISABILITY

SOCIOECONOMIC STATUS

- Lower middle class

SPIRITUAL/RELIGIOUS

- Traditional Native American spiritual beliefs

PSYCHOSOCIAL

LEGAL

ETHICAL

PRIORITIZATION

DELEGATION

PHARMACOLOGIC

- Hemabate; methylergonovine maleate (Methergine); oxytocin (Pitocin)

ALTERNATIVE THERAPY

SIGNIFICANT HISTORY

- Grand multigravida; history of preterm births; history of infant losses; history of postpartum hemorrhage

PRENATAL

Level of difficulty: Difficult

Overview: Requires background knowledge of the Native American culture and health concerns. Requires knowledge regarding asthma and asthma medications and their effects during pregnancy.

DIFFICULT

Client Profile

Ruth is a 28-year-old, married Native American, G5P2202. Ruth is a social worker on an Indian reservation in North Carolina. Her husband manages a large construction company. Her first two pregnancies occurred when she was a single teen and ended in premature births of infants at 26 and 28 weeks gestation. Both babies died from respiratory distress syndrome (RDS). Ruth was 15 years old with her first baby and 17 with the second. Ruth smoked 1 to 2 packs of cigarettes a day with her first pregnancies and did not start prenatal care until the second trimester with both of them. She was married at age 21 and had two full term pregnancies. The second two children are now one and five years old. They were both NSVD at the small birth center near the reservation. Because of Ruth's job she is well known and loved by everyone in the area. Ruth and her husband, also a Native American, are very proud of their heritage and love living near the reservation, which allows them to keep their children immersed in their culture. Ruth's grandmother is a storyteller for the tribe, and the grandchildren look forward to spending Saturday evenings with her listening to tales about Indian children. Because Ruth's work keeps her so busy she has put off starting her prenatal care for this pregnancy for several months. Although Ruth still smokes one-half pack of cigarettes a day and is overweight, she has been careful to eat properly and get adequate rest when she can.

Case Study

Today (August 15) is her initial prenatal visit at the birth center. Her last normal menstrual period (LNMP) was March 10, and she experienced some spotting on April 2. Ruth has had one minor bout of asthma since getting pregnant. (She uses an inhaler once or twice a week.) Her height is five feet two inches, and her current weight is 186 pounds. She has gained approximately 42 pounds during this pregnancy, so far. Upon examination the nurse finds her fundal height to be 29 cm. Her BP is 112/68, H&H 11.2 mg and 34%. Ruth states that this baby is very active. She has some dependent edema in both ankles. She has not experienced any headaches. She did state that her glasses don't seem to properly correct her vision these days, and the words are sometimes unclear when she tries to read. She is still experiencing some nausea and vomiting, but it is not severe. A wet mount at this visit reveals that Ruth has a vaginal candidiasis (yeast) infection. The routine labs are drawn and cultures done.

Questions

1. How many weeks gestation is Ruth at this initial visit?

2. Identify at least six high-risk factors that Ruth is presenting with.

3. Discuss Ruth's vision changes.

4. Native Americans have a higher risk for diabetes. Does Ruth present any indications of this problem?

5. During the antepartum, culture may influence what taboos and what prescriptives are needed to ensure a safe delivery (Littleton, 2001). When caring for individuals of the Native American culture the nurse should know some of the basic beliefs and behaviors that are practiced in this culture. Name four major areas where misunderstanding can occur between the non–Native American nurse and the Native American family.

6. Native Americans have higher poverty and unemployment rates than other groups of Americans. How does this affect the general health care and outcomes for Native American women?

7. Aside from diabetes, what else could account for her high fundal height?

8. Asthma is also more prevalent in the Native American population. Identify the risk associated with asthma in pregnancy.

9. Overall, how do the statistics on the Native American population compare for preterm births and teen pregnancies to other populations living in the same areas.

10. An ultrasound reveals that Ruth is carrying twins. Make a list of risks that are associated with multiple gestation pregnancies.

11. Ruth goes into preterm labor at 32 weeks gestation and delivers twin boys weighing in at 3 pounds and 2 pounds 6 ounces in the hospital. Immediately following delivery of the placenta she begins to hemorrhage. Her uterus is boggy, and the obstetrician calls for carboprost tromethamine (Hemabate) stat, while he does a bimanual compression. Is this an appropriate order for this client?

12. What would have been the immediate response if the nurse had prepared the medication and the physician had given it?

13. Name two other medications that can be used for this client that will contract the uterus.

14. List and explain at least four factors that placed Ruth at risk for this hemorrhage.

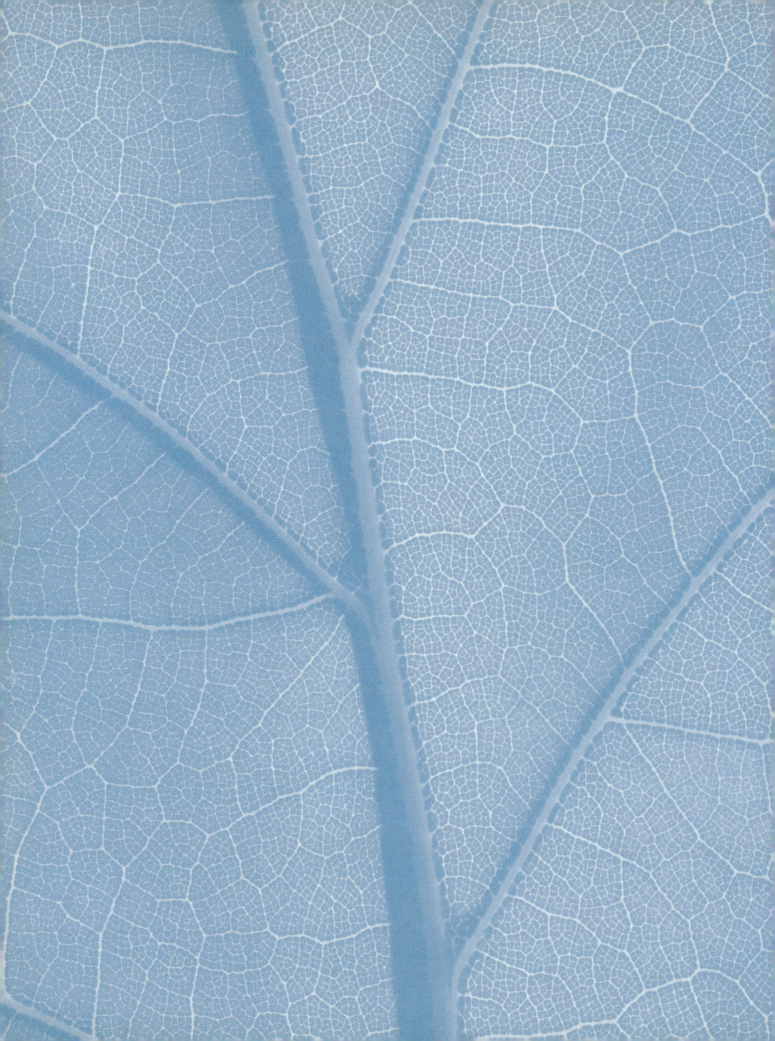

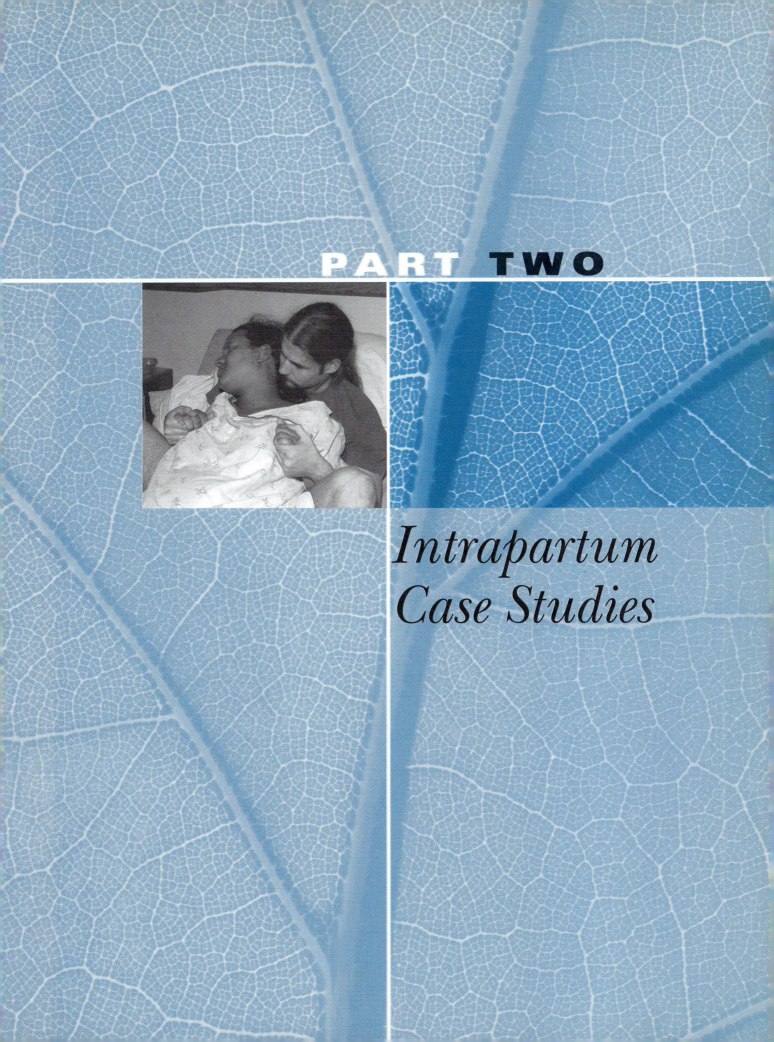

PART TWO

*Intrapartum
Case Studies*

Norma

AGE

19

SETTING

■ Certified Nurse Midwifery
office/phone triage

CULTURAL CONSIDERATIONS

■ Middle-class White American culture

ETHNICITY

■ White American

PRE-EXISTING CONDITION

CO-EXISTING CONDITION/CURRENT PROBLEMS

COMMUNICATIONS

DISABILITY

SOCIOECONOMIC STATUS

SPIRITUAL/RELIGIOUS

PSYCHOSOCIAL

LEGAL

ETHICAL

PRIORITIZATION

DELEGATION

PHARMACOLOGIC

ALTERNATIVE THERAPY

■ Aromatherapy: clary sage, jasmine, lavender, nutmeg, rose, ylang-ylang; massage

SIGNIFICANT HISTORY

■ Primigravida

INTRAPARTUM

Level of difficulty: Easy

Overview: This case requires an understanding of early labor and asks the student to use critical thinking to assess contractions and fetal well-being.

Client Profile

Norma is a 19-year-old, G1P0, MWF at 39 weeks gestation. Her pregnancy has been uneventful. Norma prides herself on having taken very good care of herself during the pregnancy. Norma is five feet three inches tall and weighs 138 pounds, having gained 22 pounds during the pregnancy.

Case Study

Norma calls her midwife's office to tell her that she has been having contractions for several hours. She tells the nurse that the baby is active, and although she cannot really rest because of the contractions, she feels she is doing very well. Norma has planned a hospital delivery with a certified nurse midwife (CNM).

Questions

1. List three questions the nurse should ask Norma at this time.

2. When should Norma be instructed to go to the hospital?

3. Norma has attended childbirth education classes. She plans to use aromatherapy, water, and massage for pain relief. How effective are these modalities in providing pain relief in labor?

4. Norma has also discussed with the certified nurse midwife (CNM) the use of intermittent fetal monitoring. Discuss the pros and cons of using continuous electronic fetal monitoring in labor.

5. Norma has also asked that she be allowed to not have an IV in labor. Her CNM has agreed to this. Discuss the pros and cons of routine IV in labor.

6. Furthermore, Norma has asked to be able to eat lightly and drink high-energy liquids in labor. Discuss the pros and cons of this.

7. Several hours later, Norma again calls the office to say that she feels she should go to the hospital. Her contractions are coming every three minutes and are lasting from one minute to 90 seconds. When she arrives at the hospital she is found to be 6 cm dilatated, completely effaced, and the baby is a +1 station. Her membranes are intact. The CNM gives her the option of having her membranes ruptured at this time (Figure 2.1). Discuss the pros and cons of this intervention.

8. The nurse is checking the fetus and Norma's contractions intermittently. How often should they be assessed?

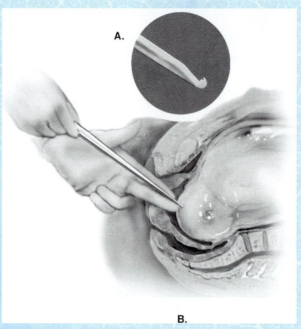

Figure 2.1   *Artificial rupture of membranes (AROM).*

9. How are contractions assessed in labor?

10. After two hours of continued strong contractions Norma is completely effaced and 10 cm dilatated. Norma says she is tired, doesn't feel like pushing, and wants to rest prior to pushing. Discuss the pros and cons of allowing her to rest at this time.

Holly

AGE

29

SETTING

- Home

CULTURAL CONSIDERATIONS

ETHNICITY

- White American

PRE-EXISTING CONDITION

- Blindness

CO-EXISTING CONDITION/CURRENT PROBLEMS

- Postdate

COMMUNICATIONS

- Client is blind

DISABILITY

- Blindness

SOCIOECONOMIC STATUS

- Upper middle class

SPIRITUAL/RELIGIOUS

PSYCHOSOCIAL

- Extended family support

LEGAL

ETHICAL

PRIORITIZATION

DELEGATION

PHARMACOLOGIC

ALTERNATIVE THERAPY

SIGNIFICANT HISTORY

- Primigravida; auto accident causing blindness

INTRAPARTUM

Level of difficulty: Easy

Overview: This case looks at the difference between a post-date and a post-mature fetus. It explores the advantage of home birth for a client with sensory deprivation, i.e., a blind client.

Client Profile

Holly is a 29-year-old, blind, G1P0, MWF at 41 weeks gestation. Holly is an attorney for the state family and children's division and is now on maternity leave. Holly lost her sight 13 years ago as a result of a head injury in an auto accident. She is an extremely determined individual and finished high school after her accident, went on to a community college, became a paralegal, got her criminal justice degree, and finally completed law school. It took her a little longer than most individuals but she graduated with honors. She met her husband in law school and they have been happily married for two years. She did her internship at the Division of Children and Families for the state and they were so impressed by her abilities that they hired her right after graduation. Holly's 14-year-old sister moved in with her two years ago. Both of their parents were killed in the accident that blinded Holly. Until two years ago her sister had been living with an aunt. She and her sister are very close, and the sister cannot wait until the baby is born so she can help care for him. Holly's pregnancy has progressed normally. All of her lab work is wnl. The baby is in a cephalic presentation. Last week Holly's midwife ordered a NST, which was reactive. Holly has also been doing daily fetal movement counts, and they have demonstrated an active healthy baby.

Case Study

Holly is in active labor at home at 41-2/7 weeks gestation. She wants a home birth since she feels that she will be in familiar surroundings and feel more in control. Two midwives have been with Holly for the past three hours monitoring her baby and contractions. She is now 8 cm, 100% effaced, and +1 station. Holly's husband and sister have been wonderful support for her. During the contractions they take turns dancing with Holly, and even though she is in transition she responds positively to their support and gets relief by the movement. The baby's heart rate is in the 140s with good long-term variability. There are no decelerations, and there are occasional accelerations. Holly's water breaks with a large gush. The fluid is clear without any odor.

Questions

1. What are the advantages for Holly in a home birth?

2. What coping mechanisms is Holly using to deal with the contractions? Why are these particularly good for Holly?

3. In general, discuss the safety of a planned home birth.

4. Why did the midwife order a non-stress test (NST) last week? What is the significance of a reactive NST?

5. What other test might she have ordered? Why?

6. What are the possible consequences of a pregnancy continuing past the established date (postdate)?

7. What is the most important nursing action after the rupture of the membranes?

8. Holly continued to eat lightly and drink fluids throughout her labor. Discuss the safety of this.

9. Describe the fetal heart pattern.

10. How are fetal heart tones (FHTs) monitored without an electronic fetal monitor at home?

11. Holly delivers a baby boy after 45 minutes of pushing in a squatting position over an intact perineum. The baby's APGARS are 9 and 10. She then immediately puts the baby to breast. Discuss the squatting position for pushing.

12. What is the advantage of not cutting an episiotomy?

13. The midwife does not cut the cord immediately, but places the baby on her mom and waits for the cord to stop pulsating. What are the advantages and disadvantages of this action?

14. Aside from the benefits of the quality of the breast milk, what is the particular advantage for Holly of breastfeeding?

Leticia

AGE

15

SETTING

■ Hospital urgent care center

CULTURAL CONSIDERATIONS

■ Puerto Rican traditional beliefs

ETHNICITY

■ Hispanic American

PRE-EXISTING CONDITION

■ Obesity

CO-EXISTING CONDITION/CURRENT PROBLEM

■ Precipitous delivery

COMMUNICATIONS

DISABILITY

SOCIOECONOMIC STATUS

SPIRITUAL/RELIGIOUS

PSYCHOSOCIAL

■ Denial of pregnancy; no identified fob

LEGAL

■ Minor

ETHICAL

PRIORITIZATION

■ Immediate care of baby and mother after a precipitous birth

DELEGATION

PHARMACOLOGIC

ALTERNATIVE THERAPY

SIGNIFICANT HISTORY

■ Primigravida

INTRAPARTUM

Level of difficulty: Easy

Overview: This case requires an understanding of adolescent behavior. It also requires critical thinking concerning legal implications regarding care of a pregnant minor.

Client Profile

Leticia is a 15-year-old, G1P0, SHF at 36-4/7 wga. She is visiting her sister in Florida (from Michigan) for a three-day weekend to get a break from the cold weather. Leticia is five feet two inches tall and weighs 168 pounds; she wears baggy clothes and is in complete denial of her pregnancy. Her parents, first-generation Puerto Rican immigrants (in Michigan), and sister are totally unaware that she is pregnant. Because of her denial, she has had no prenatal care.

Case Study

At 1 a.m. the night after her arrival in Florida, Leticia begins to get strong stomach "cramps." She does not tell her sister until they have gone on for most of the night. Finally, at 7 a.m. she wakes her sister in tears and tells her about "this awful stomachache," she has. Her sister immediately decides to take her to the nearest urgent care center for treatment. Because she is only 15, she is admitted to the pediatric area of the center and immediately taken to an exam room because she is doubled over in pain. She has continued to wear her usual baggy sweat suit and has not yet faced up to the fact that she is pregnant. Five minutes after being put into the exam room the nurse enters to get her vital signs and take an assessment of her problem. The physician is just finishing suturing a small child's hand in the room next door. It takes the nurse about two minutes to realize what is happening. She barely has a chance to put on gloves to do an internal exam when Leticia begins to push hard and her membranes rupture. Within five minutes the nurse delivers a four-pound baby girl with APGARS of 9 and 10, who is screaming and pink. From examination the baby appears to be between 35 and 36 weeks gestation.

Questions

1. During a precipitous birth, what are the priorities for the baby?

2. What are the priorities for the mother?

3. Identify three OSHA concerns in this situation.

4. Is it possible for any woman to completely deny a pregnancy that goes nearly to term?

5. Is there any problem with Leticia receiving care as a minor without her parents present?

6. Who is the legal guardian of the baby?

7. What are the nursing priorities for the immediate postpartum?

8. How will the nurse prepare Leticia for her discharge with her baby?

9. Leticia still denies she ever had sex. How will the father be listed on the birth certificate?

10. Should the nurse suggest that Leticia breastfeed her baby?

Lydia

AGE

23

SETTING

■ Private OB practice/hospital

CULTURAL CONSIDERATIONS

■ Traditional Colombian culture

ETHNICITY

■ Colombian

PRE-EXISTING CONDITION

■ Healthy female w/normal term pregnancy

CO-EXISTING CONDITION/CURRENT PROBLEM

COMMUNICATIONS

■ Non-English-speaking client

DISABILITY

SOCIOECONOMIC STATUS

■ Affluent

SPIRITUAL/RELIGIOUS

PSYCHOSOCIAL

LEGAL

ETHICAL

■ Cultural beliefs vs safety

PRIORITIZATION

DELEGATION

PHARMACOLOGIC

■ Epidural anesthesia

ALTERNATIVE THERAPY

SIGNIFICANT HISTORY

■ Primigravida

INTRAPARTUM

Level of difficulty: Easy

Overview: This case requires the learner to assess safety factors when they conflict with cultural practices.

Client Profile

Lydia is a 23-year-old, G1P0, MHF from Colombia visiting her sister in Miami, Florida. She does not speak English. She had only intended to visit her sister for a few weeks; however, political events in Colombia have made it impossible for her to return home. She has now been here two months and is 38 weeks gestation. She made an appointment at a private OB/CNM service to discuss her delivery. She did not bring her records since she never intended to be here this long. An initial OB visit is performed including all labs. Her sister is her interpreter. In Colombia, Lydia has already discussed with her obstetrician that she desires to have an elective cesarean section. She is from a prominent wealthy political family and considers vaginal delivery primitive and disgusting.

Case Study

Her initial prenatal visit reveals a healthy, 23-year-old, G1P0, MHF with a normally progressing intrauterine pregnancy (IUP) at 38 weeks gestational age. Her fundal height is 38 cm, there is positive fetal movement, the heart tones are in the LLQ in the 140s, all of her urine is negative, her VS are normal with a BP of 110/70, and she has no edema or headaches. Her personal and family history is benign. Her pelvis is gynecoid and adequate with blunt spines and pubic arch of over 90 degrees. Baby's estimated weight at this time is around six and a half pounds. As she is leaving, the nurse tells her that she needs to come back in one week. Her sister relays this to her and she seems upset. She tells her sister that she thought that she would be checking into the hospital for her cesarean section tonight.

Questions

1. What are the compared risks to the mother and the infant in a cesarean section versus vaginal delivery?

2. How should the nurse approach this situation?

3. Having a cesarean section is obviously a cultural norm for Lydia. At what point do respecting culture and the risk of compromising safe care begin to conflict? How do you prioritize this dilemma?

4. List at least three arguments that Lydia might use to justify her desire for a cesarean section. How should the nurse reply to each?

5. What are the possibilities that, if Lydia were to go into labor, she would still deliver by a cesarean section?

6. Are they increased over another woman who does not desire a cesarean section?

7. Lydia, against her wishes, is given an appointment to come back at 39 weeks. She tells her sister in Spanish, "This country is so backward. I would never have to tolerate this pregnancy this long back home." She then begins to cry. The sister explains this to the nurse. How should the nurse reply?

8. The nurse would like to offer Lydia some classes on labor preparation. How might this sensitive topic be approached?

9. At the 39-week visit, Lydia is obviously angry and again, through her sister, she insists on ending this pregnancy tonight with a cesarean section. "Why do they make me suffer so?" She asks her sister who interprets for the nurse. It is obvious that Lydia is used to getting her own way. Her BP is 148/76; FHTs at the left lower quadrant (LLQ) are in the 150s. She has lost two pounds in the past week and states that the baby is not moving as much as before. The obstetrician orders an NST that is reactive. Her Bishop score is 8. He also offers to induce her with an epidural if she wishes. Explain the BP elevation and weight loss. She accepts the induction if "I will not feel any pain."

10. What is a Bishop score?

11. Six hours into the labor with the epidural, Lydia has only dilated to 4 cm, is 100% effaced, and at zero station. She delivers via a cesarean section for failure to progress (FTP). Discuss this outcome.

Kathleen

AGE

21

SETTING

- Freestanding birth center

CULTURAL CONSIDERATIONS

ETHNICITY

- White American

PRE-EXISTING CONDITION

CO-EXISTING CONDITION/CURRENT PROBLEM

- R/o breech presentation

COMMUNICATIONS

- Deaf client

DISABILITY

- Deafness

SOCIOECONOMIC STATUS

SPIRITUAL/RELIGIOUS

- Christian Scientist

PSYCHOSOCIAL

LEGAL

ETHICAL

PRIORITIZATION

DELEGATION

PHARMACOLOGIC

ALTERNATIVE THERAPY

SIGNIFICANT HISTORY

- Multigravida

MODERATE

INTRAPARTUM

Level of difficulty: Moderate

Overview: Requires assessing a client for malpresentation and to rule out labor. Looks at communications with a deaf client.

Client Profile

Kathleen is a deaf, 21-year-old, G2P1001, MWF at 38 weeks gestational age. Kathleen has had a normal pregnancy throughout. She is very happy about the pregnancy and excited about the coming birth.

Case Study

Kathleen reports to the freestanding birth center at 1 a.m. with her husband, complaining of cramping for the past four hours and a vaginal discharge. Vital signs are: fetal heart tones (FHT) 140s, located just above and left of the umbilicus, with several accelerations heard while auscultating for two minutes, good fetal movement (FM); T 98°F, P 76, R 18, BP 110/68; contractions palpated every three minutes lasting 50 to 60 seconds and of moderate intensity with good resting tone. Her vaginal exam (VE) reveals 4 cm dilated and 80% effaced.

Questions

1. What questions does the nurse need to ask Kathleen to assess her contractions?

2. How do true labor contractions feel to the woman, as opposed to Braxton-Hicks contractions?

3. What is the significance of the FHT?

4. What further information is needed from the vaginal exam (VE) to assess her condition?

5. What is the significance of the vaginal discharge?

6. How will the nurse check to see if the membranes have ruptured?

7. If the baby were not engaged, would it pose a problem at this stage of labor?

8. What is the significance of the fact that she is deaf?

9. What is the best way for the nurse to communicate with Kathleen since she is deaf?

10. What is the significance if Kathleen's membranes are ruptured and meconium is present?

11. If Kathleen is in active labor, will she be allowed to deliver in the freestanding birth center?

Cassandra

AGE

24

SETTING

- Birth center to hospital transfer

CULTURAL CONSIDERATIONS

- Black-Muslim traditions

ETHNICITY

- Black American

PRE-EXISTING CONDITION

- Short stature

CO-EXISTING CONDITION/CURRENT PROBLEM

- Shoulder dystocia; GBS positive; FTP

COMMUNICATIONS

DISABILITY

SOCIOECONOMIC STATUS

SPIRITUAL/RELIGIOUS

PSYCHOSOCIAL

LEGAL

ETHICAL

PRIORITIZATION

DELEGATION

PHARMACOLOGIC

- Ampicillin; oxytocin (Pitocin)

ALTERNATIVE THERAPY

SIGNIFICANT HISTORY

- Multigravida

MODERATE

INTRAPARTUM

Level of difficulty: Moderate

Overview: Requires critical thinking to assess and identify treatment for shoulder dystocia.

Client Profile

Cassandra is a 24-year-old, G3P1011, MBF. She is five feet tall and her current weight at 40 weeks gestation is 142 pounds. Her pre-pregnant weight was 125 pounds. After 16 hours of active labor and being 6 cm, 100% effaced, and −2 station for six hours, she is transported from her planned home birth to the hospital. She is GBS positive and at the time of transport has already received two doses of ampicillin 1 gram each, six hours apart, by IV. Her membranes have been ruptured (SROM) for two hours. On admission to the labor unit her BP is 110/78, T 98.4, P 72, R 20. Contractions are q 5 to 6 minutes, lasting from 50 to 60 seconds, and strong at the peak (by palpation). The mother is having good relaxation between contractions. The FHT are reassuring with occasional accelerations: baseline of 130s to 140s and both long-term and short-term variability present. There are no decelerations. The estimated fetal weight (EFW) is 8 pounds. Her last baby was 7 pounds 10 ounces and was a normal spontaneous vaginal delivery (NSVD) at home with a licensed Muslim midwife. The baby is in a cephalic presentation left occiput anterior presentation (LOA). Reason for transfer: Maternal fatigue with failure to progress (FTP) in the last six hours with adequate contractions, which in the past three hours were becoming farther apart and weaker.

The obstetrician orders:

1. Pitocin IV to be increased every 20 minutes until contractions are coming every 2 to 3 minutes and lasting 90 seconds
2. Continue ampicillin 1 gram every 6 hours until delivery
3. Intrauterine pressure catheter (IUPC) and fetal scalp electrode (FSE) (Figure 2.2).

Case Study

Two hours following admission her contractions are every two minutes, strong, and 90 seconds in duration. Cassandra has requested an epidural anesthesia and is now resting.

The nurse notes the following at this time:

BP 100/60

Temperature 99

Pulse 82

Respirations 20

Vaginal exam (VE) 8 cm, 100%, −2 station

FHT 150s no accelerations, minimal variability, no decelerations, baby is moving during rest periods between contractions

Uterus is relaxed between contractions

A foley catheter has been inserted and output is sufficient

Figure 2.2 *Placement of an intrauterine pressure catheter and fetal scalp electrode.*

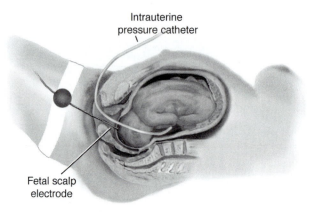

Intrauterine pressure catheter

Fetal scalp electrode

Questions

1. What is the significance of the baby still being at a negative 2 station?

2. Assess the following data: FHT 150s, no accelerations, minimal variability, no decelerations, baby is moving during rest periods between contractions.

3. What is the rationale for the ampicillin?

4. Cassandra had desired a natural home birth with no pain medications. What factors led up to her requesting an epidural?

5. Two hours later she is totally effaced and 10 cm dilated (complete, complete). With encouragement, she pushed for two hours and managed to push the head out. Immediately the head turtles. What does the term *turtle* mean?

6. What are the causes of shoulder dystocia (Figure 2.3)?

7. What position should the nurse assist Cassandra into in order to assist the obstetrician in the delivery of the shoulders? (List two possible positions that may be helpful at this time and explain why they can help.)

8. Distinguish between supra pubic pressure and fundal pressure (Figure 2.4).

9. Which one will help to deliver the shoulders and why?

10. What measures should the nurse take to prepare for immediate care of this newborn?

11. What possible injuries might this baby sustain as a result of this delivery?

12. What injuries might the mother sustain?

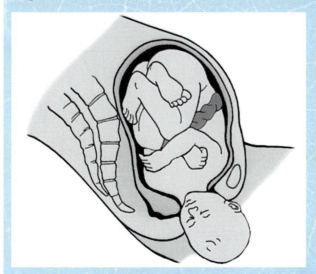

Figure 2.3   *Shoulder dystocia.*

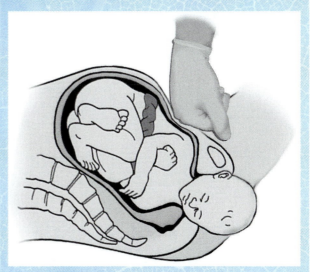

Figure 2.4   *Supra pubic pressure to release shoulder dystocia.*

Mimi

AGE

36

SETTING

- Hospital labor and delivery unit

CULTURAL CONSIDERATIONS

ETHNICITY

- Indonesian American

PRE-EXISTING CONDITION

CO-EXISTING CONDITION/CURRENT PROBLEM

- No prenatal care; moderate meconium staining

COMMUNICATIONS

DISABILITY

SOCIOECONOMIC STATUS

SPIRITUAL/RELIGIOUS

- Hindu

PSYCHOSOCIAL

LEGAL

ETHICAL

PRIORITIZATION

DELEGATION

PHARMACOLOGIC

ALTERNATIVE THERAPY

SIGNIFICANT HISTORY

- Multigravida

MODERATE

INTRAPARTUM

Level of difficulty: Moderate

Overview: This case requires using critical thinking to identify factors that interfere with normal fetal descent and identification of interventions to assist the infant to descend. It also requires identification of fetal heart tone patterns that indicate stress and abnormal contraction patterns.

Client Profile

Mimi is a 36-year-old, married, G3P2002, Indonesian female. This is her third pregnancy in three years. Like many Indonesian couples, she and her husband decided to put off having children until they had established their careers. She did not have prenatal care, and her due date is uncertain. Her fundal height is 36 cm. She is five feet six inches tall, and her current weight is 168 pounds.

Case Study

Mimi arrives at the hospital, with her sister and mother, in active labor. Her husband is with her but it is her mother and sister who assist her. She is admitted through the emergency room. She was 6 cm, 100% effaced; and the baby is at −1 station at the time of admission. Her membranes are ruptured, and the fluid is moderately meconium stained.

Questions

1. Shortly after Mimi is admitted to the labor suite she starts to push. The nurse checks her and finds that she is 7 cm and still at −1 station. What problems can result from Mimi's pushing at this time in the labor?

2. How can the nurse help Mimi stop pushing at this time?

3. What is the significance of the meconium in the fluid?

4. What special preparations will the nurse make to care for this infant immediately after birth?

5. The baby's head is in anterior asynclitism. What factors may account for this position?

6. The head engages. What problems can occur if the baby remains in a persistent asynclitic presentation?

7. What can be done to help direct the fetal head into the pelvis and convert the head to a synclitic presentation?

8. Three hours after admission the nurse notes that the baby's head is beginning to form a large caput. Fetal heart tones are noted to decrease to 110 bmp around the height of the contractions and return to the baseline of 130s just prior to the end of the contractions. What is the significance of these observations?

9. Bloody show is increasing and Mimi has an increased urge to push. The nurse checks her and finds that she has an anterior cervical lip. What might the nurse do to help reduce the lip and prepare Mimi to deliver?

10. After the lip is reduced, the baby begins to descend rapidly. The infant is crowning and the heart tones fall to 90s. The physician is preparing to deliver the head in the next few contractions. Identify two nursing actions that are appropriate at this time.

Danielle

AGE

41

SETTING

- Hospital labor and delivery unit

CULTURAL CONSIDERATIONS

ETHNICITY

- White American

PRE-EXISTING CONDITION

CO-EXISTING CONDITION/CURRENT PROBLEM

- AMA; older primigravida; augmentation; FTP; variable decelerations

COMMUNICATIONS

DISABILITY

SOCIOECONOMIC STATUS

SPIRITUAL/RELIGIOUS

PSYCHOSOCIAL

LEGAL

ETHICAL

PRIORITIZATION

DELEGATION

PHARMACOLOGIC

- Oxytocin (Pitocin)

ALTERNATIVE THERAPY

- Chinese medicine; Yongquan; Hoku; kidney 1; large intestine 4

SIGNIFICANT HISTORY

- Primigravida

MODERATE

INTRAPARTUM

Level of difficulty: Moderate

Overview: Requires assessing the pros and cons of induction and examination of the effects of interventions used to induce and augment labor.

Client Profile

Danielle is a 41-year-old, G1P0, MWF, who has experienced a normal pregnancy. She is five feet three inches tall and her current weight is 148 pounds. Danielle works as a bartender and due to the long hours on her feet she has experienced +2 pitting edema in both ankles. The swelling goes down when she lies down. Last week she told the nurse that she felt foolish because she had had a crazy dream where she thought she was giving birth to a litter of puppies. Afterwards she sighed and said, "I'm too old to be going through all of this."

Case Study

Danielle arrived at the hospital on Friday afternoon complaining of intermittent mild to moderate contractions for the past 12 hours. She denied ruptured membranes and bleeding. She is 39 weeks gestation. In the triage exam she was found to be 60% effaced, 1 cm dilatated, and −3 station. Her membranes were intact. Her contractions were 5 to 6 minutes apart, lasting one minute, and strong at the peak. The obstetrician decided to admit her to the labor and delivery suite and to artificially rupture her membranes (AROM) and begin Pitocin to augment her labor. Seven hours after her admission she was diagnosed with failure to progress (FTP). She had dilated to 2 cm and 100% effaced station −3 after six hours of Pitocin-augmented labor and an epidural. She was given internal fetal heart monitoring/internal uterine monitoring, which indicated a fetal heart rate baseline of 120 to 126 bpm with occasional accelerations for the first two hours. For the last hour of the labor she had a baseline of 140 to 142 bpm and an increasing number of variable decelerations. These decelerations stopped when she was placed on her right side. She was given a cesarean section. Her baby girl weighed 8 pounds and was 21 inches long. Her APGARS were 8 at one minute and 8 at five minutes with points taken off for tone and color.

Questions

1. Is there any significance to the fact that Danielle is 41 years old?

2. Is there any significance to the fact that this is her first pregnancy?

3. Discuss Danielle's dreams.

4. What is the significance of the +2 pitting edema in her ankles?

5. What are the advantages or disadvantages of cesarean section following labor as opposed to scheduled cesarean section?

6. List the indications and risk of artificial rupture of membranes (AROM).

7. Why do you think a cesarean section was done?

8. What is the difference between Pitocin induction and Pitocin augmentation?

9. Analyze the information given regarding the fetal heart tones.

10. Why did the variable decelerations stop after the client was positioned on her right side? What other positions might have been used?

11. What effect might having an epidural have had on this labor and the cesarean section outcome?

12. What else might have been done to help the baby descend and labor progress?

Josie

AGE	SPIRITUAL/RELIGIOUS
26	■ Episcopal
SETTING	**PSYCHOSOCIAL**
■ Birth center	
CULTURAL CONSIDERATIONS	**LEGAL**
■ American urban professional culture	
ETHNICITY	**ETHICAL**
■ White American	
PRE-EXISTING CONDITION	**PRIORITIZATION**
CO-EXISTING CONDITION/CURRENT PROBLEMS	**DELEGATION**
■ Prolapsed cord	
COMMUNICATIONS	**PHARMACOLOGIC**
DISABILITY	**ALTERNATIVE THERAPY**
SOCIOECONOMIC STATUS	**SIGNIFICANT HISTORY**
■ Professional	■ Multigravida

MODERATE

INTRAPARTUM

Level of difficulty: Moderate

Overview: This case requires identification of risk factors associated with a prolapsed cord. It also requires that the student identify the appropriate emergency care required when a prolapsed cord occurs.

Client Profile

Josie is a 26-year-old, G2P1001, MWF. Her pregnancy has been uneventful. She and her husband are very happy about this pregnancy. Their first child is three years old. Josie is a secondary school math teacher. She has remained employed throughout the pregnancy until last week when voiding frequency and urgency, and shortness of breath became such problems that she decided to take a leave until after the baby is born. They plan to deliver at the birth center where their first child was born. Josie's pregnancy is at 38 weeks gestation. She was just seen in the office this morning, and she and baby were doing well. The urine chemstrip was negative; BP and FHT were normal. The baby was at a −1 to −2 station, and her cervix was 80% effaced and 2 cm dilatated. Josie had lost two pounds since last week. She had no edema and no headaches or vision changes. At that time she was not experiencing any contractions.

Case Study

At 1 a.m. Josie and her husband call the midwife to tell her that Josie's waters have broken, and they are going to the birth center. When the midwife greets them Josie is smiling and relaxed. She has been having contractions for about four hours at home, and they are just beginning to get strong. The baby is active. Immediately upon getting to the birth center Josie asks to use the toilet. As soon as she sits down she tells the midwife that something is coming out of her vagina. The midwife recognizes a prolapsed cord (Figure 2.5).

Figure 2.5 *Prolapsed cord.*

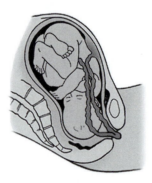

Questions

1. The midwife calls the nurse to assist in positioning Josie. What position will they place her in?

2. What are the risks associated with prolapsed cord?

3. What factors contributed to the cord prolapsing?

4. While the midwife does a vaginal exam, the nurse checks the fetal heart tones. What patterns might the nurse expect to hear?

5. What other immediate actions are needed at this time?

6. Should the cord be replaced into the vagina?

7. Josie is to be transported to the hospital. How should this transport be accomplished?

8. At the hospital Josie is given an emergency cesarean section. (It is less than 30 minutes since she first entered the birth center.) The baby's APGARS are 2 at one minute, 5 at five minutes, and then 6 at ten minutes. The baby is put on a ventilator and admitted to the neonatal intensive care unit. Within eight hours the baby is able to be removed from the ventilator and is doing well. What problems can be anticipated for this baby?

9. What problems might the mother experience postpartum?

Jennifer

AGE

17

SETTING

- Hospital labor and delivery unit

CULTURAL CONSIDERATIONS

- Black American

ETHNICITY

- Black American

PRE-EXISTING CONDITION

CO-EXISTING CONDITION/CURRENT PROBLEM

- Preterm labor with spontaneous rupture of membranes (SROM)

COMMUNICATIONS

DISABILITY

SOCIOECONOMIC STATUS

- Low income

SPIRITUAL/RELIGIOUS

PSYCHOSOCIAL

LEGAL

- Minor

ETHICAL

PRIORITIZATION

DELEGATION

PHARMACOLOGIC

ALTERNATIVE THERAPY

- Transcutaneous electrical stimulation (TENS); sterile water papules

SIGNIFICANT HISTORY

- Primigravida

INTRAPARTUM

Level of difficulty: Difficult

Overview: This case requires that students be able to visualize the rotation of the fetus to identify problems with OP presentations. Students need to have knowledge of the role of the doula as well as knowledge of comfort measures. Furthermore, they must identify when labor stimulation is and is not appropriate. It requires them to determine how appropriate pain medication is in the later part of active labor, means of determining ROM, and assessment of labor progress.

DIFFICULT

Client Profile

Jennifer is a 17-year-old, G1P0, MBF. Jennifer is an active high school senior. She attended childbirth classes held at her high school. She attends a special program for pregnant teens. She has been careful to eat well and avoid all hazards that might harm her baby. She is looking forward to holding her baby and does not appear to be afraid of the coming labor.

Case Study

Jennifer is admitted in active labor at 36-2/7 weeks gestation. She has been experiencing contractions for the past six hours. For the past two hours they have been getting stronger and lasting up to one minute each. She believes that her membranes may have ruptured. She is accompanied by her husband, her mother, and a doula. Upon examination, the nurse determines that she is 3 cm dilatated; 90% effaced, and at a station of −3. The baby's heart tones are 120s with no decelerations. The nurse confirms that her membranes have ruptured spontaneously (SROM). According to Jennifer this occurred two hours ago. Contractions are one minute in length, q 5 minutes, strong with good relaxation between contractions.

Questions

1. What is the role of the doula?

2. How did the nurse determine if Jennifer's membranes have ruptured?

3. What is the significance of the findings from the pelvic exam?

4. What is the significance of the ruptured membranes in Jennifer's case?

5. What stage of labor is she in?

After six hours Jennifer is 5 cm, 100% effaced, and −3 station. The nurse notes that the baby is in an occiput posterior (OP) presentation. This presentation puts the hard back of the baby's head against the mother's spine. Descent is slower and more painful.

6. How does the baby's presentation impact the labor?

7. What comfort measures might the doula use to help Jennifer cope with the labor?

8. What positions might the mother use to help the baby rotate and descend?

Four hours later the mother is 8 cm, 100% effaced, and −2 station. The baby has rotated to the left occiput transverse (LOT) presentation. This turns the baby to face the mother's side and reduces the pressure on her back.

9. Jennifer complains that she needs to push. What are the consequences if she were to push at this point?

Jennifer does not progress in the next two hours, the baby is developing a large caput, and the FHT are now 150s with an occasional variable deceleration. Contractions are every two minutes, 90 seconds in length, and strong with good relaxation between. The obstetrician expresses concern that he may need to do a cesarean section. Jennifer asks for more time to see if she can begin to progress again.

10. Which of the following would be appropriate management of Jennifer at this point?

a. The doctor allows her two more hours to dilatate and orders Pitocin to make the contraction more effective.

b. She is given an epidural to help the baby rotate and descend.

c. She is given meperidine (Demerol) 50 mg for pain to help her relax.

d. Jennifer is given IV antibiotics.

e. The doula helps Jennifer assume a hands-and-knees position.

Multiple Clients

SETTING

- Hospital labor unit

CULTURAL CONSIDERATIONS

ETHNICITY

- Varied

PRE-EXISTING CONDITION

CO-EXISTING CONDITION/CURRENT PROBLEM

- Meconium stained fluid

COMMUNICATIONS

DISABILITY

SPIRITUAL/RELIGIOUS

PSYCHOSOCIAL

LEGAL

- Need for nursing supervisor to be notified of increased staffing needs and inability to contact MD

ETHICAL

PRIORITIZATION

- Delayed starting epidural anesthesia without ability to monitor client for potential complication

DELEGATION

- Responsibility that can be given to the labor room technician

PHARMACOLOGIC

- Epidural; oxytocin (Pitocin)

ALTERNATIVE THERAPY

INTRAPARTUM

Level of difficulty: Difficult

Overview: This case involves asking the student to look at staffing in a very busy labor unit and to prioritize care based on immediate need. Four laboring mothers are presented who are all in need of nursing care from two RNs and a technician. The student is expected to identify the need for going outside the unit to seek assistance from the nursing supervisor and placing a call to any OB in the house when the physician is delayed in transit to the hospital. The student is also expected to be assertive in not allowing interventions with potential adverse effects to be done until adequate nursing staff can be assigned.

DIFFICULT

Unit Profile

Mt. St. Vincent Hospital is a 300-bed general hospital. The maternity unit is a level I. There are four beds in the labor unit and an early labor lounge. It is 11:30 p.m., and the second shift just came on duty.

Case Study

There are three clients already admitted in labor. The first client admitted to the unit is Jeanette, a 26-year-old SWF, primigravida at 41 weeks gestation. She was admitted three hours ago at 100% effacement and 3 cm dilatated. The baby is at zero station. Her membranes are intact.

The second client in labor is Frances, a 39-year-old married Haitian American multigravida who was admitted yesterday morning with preterm, premature rupture of membranes at 36 weeks gestation. She is being induced with Pitocin and her last vaginal exam was done at 11:15 p.m. She had progressed to 6 cm, 100% effaced; and the baby is at +2 station. Her vital signs at 11:00 p.m. were temperature 100.2, pulse 88, respirations 24, and BP 130/88.

The third client is Ida, a 17-year-old SWF, primigravida who was admitted two hours ago after being in labor at home all day. Two hours ago a vaginal exam (VE) revealed that she was 6 cm, 100% effaced; and the baby was at +1 station. Her membranes broke earlier in the day at home.

Questions

1. There are two RNs and one labor technician on duty tonight. While change of shift report was being given the following requests from the women were received at the nurses' station. At 11:30 p.m.:

1. Frances is asking for an epidural.
2. Jeanette wants to take off the electronic fetal monitor and walk around.
3. Ida wants to get up and use the bathroom.

There is also a call from admitting that a new client has just arrived and needs to be brought to the labor unit. The labor unit is expected to send someone to transport her. The clerk at the admission desk said that she seems to be in very active labor. This is her fourth baby.

Which clients need the most immediate attention?

2. At 11:50 p.m. while walking around in her room, Jeanette's membranes rupture. The fluid is dark greenish with particles in it. It also has a foul odor. When the nurse checks the baby's heart rate she hears an increase in the fetal heart tones prior to a contraction, a sharp drop, and then a rapid return with the heart tones going above the baseline for a few seconds after the contraction. Describe the nursing actions that are appropriate at this time and give the rationales for each.

3. Ida complains that she needs to have a bowel movement. She is irritable and refuses to continue her breathing with her doula. Her legs are shaking and she feels nauseated and begins to vomit. The nurse knows that these are all signs of what?

4. The new client is Julie, a multigravida admitted to the labor unit at 12 midnight. She is found to be 100% effaced, 9 cm dilatated; and the baby is at +3 station. She tells the nurse that she feels the urge to push. She is also demanding pain medication. How should the nurse respond to this client?

5. At 12:05 a.m. Ida is checked by one of the RNs and found to be 10 cm dilatated, 100% effaced; and the baby is at +1 station. The fetal heart tones are 130s with accelerations and no decelerations. She says she is tired and does not feel like pushing. What nursing actions are needed at this time?

6. Describe the best use of the staffing at 12:10 a.m.

7. At 12:20 a.m. the technician notifies the RN that Jeanette's fetal heart tones have decreased to 90 bmp for the past one minute and have not returned to the baseline. The nurse has instructed the technician to turn her to her side and start her on oxygen. A call was placed to her doctor 20 minutes ago when her membranes ruptured and meconium was noted. The physician has not returned the call as yet. The fetal heart tones do not improve when she is placed on her side. What nursing actions are required at this time?

8. The nurse anesthetist arrives to do the epidural for Frances at 12:30 a.m. The anesthetist tells the nurse that she has to get back to surgery as soon as possible and wants to quickly get the epidural started. Prior to the epidural being given, what nursing care needs to be completed?

9. At 12:25 a.m. Jeanette's physican calls. He is on his way to the hospital but is caught in a traffic jam and will be there within 15 minutes. He tells the nurse to have Jeanette prepared for a cesarean section and then to notify the surgical area to prepare for her.

What nursing actions need to be done to prepare her for surgery?

10. Prior to the epidural being started Frances complains about the need to push. The nurse checks her and finds her to be only 8 cm dilatated. What would the consequences be if she started to push at this time?

Margaret

AGE

22

SETTING

- Hospital labor and delivery unit

CULTURAL CONSIDERATIONS

- Accepts American medicalization concepts of pregnancy and birth

ETHNICITY

- Black American

PRE-EXISTING CONDITION

CO-EXISTING CONDITION/CURRENT PROGRAM

- Amniotic fluid embolism; placental abruption; disseminated intravascular coagulopathy (DIC)

COMMUNICATIONS

DISABILITY

SOCIOECONOMIC STATUS

- Lower middle class

SPIRITUAL/RELIGIOUS

PSYCHOSOCIAL

LEGAL

ETHICAL

PRIORITIZATION

- CPR; client needs in an emergency

DELEGATION

PHARMACOLOGIC

ALTERNATIVE THERAPY

SIGNIFICANT HISTORY

- Multigravida

INTRAPARTUM

Level of difficulty: Difficult

Overview: This case requires recognition of an amniotic fluid embolism with development of DIC during a normal labor, nursing assessment of client condition, and prioritizing nursing care in an emergency delivery.

Client Profile

Margaret is a 22-year-old, MBF who recently moved to Georgia from Detroit. She is a G3P2002 and currently at 38 wga. Margaret started prenatal care at 8 weeks gestation. She is five feet four inches tall and her current weight is 130 pounds. Her total weight gain thus far is 18 pounds. She works as a telemarketer 10 hours a day, 5 days a week. She eats fast foods but loves to snack on raw vegetables. Her last baby was born five years ago, full term, and without complications. She was not happy about the birth but endured it, and now is feeling apprehensive about this coming birth. She just wants it over with so that she can get on with her life. Her husband plans to stay with her in labor as does her mother and a sister. She has decided to get an epidural (she had one last time) as soon as the labor becomes "too much to handle."

Case Study

Margaret is being seen today at the prenatal clinic because of a complaint of decreased fetal movement. A biophysical profile reveals a healthy baby with good tone, movement, adequate amniotic fluid, breathing movements, and a reactive non-stress test. The baby is estimated to be approximately 7 pounds. Her first baby was 6 pounds 9 ounces. Her cervix is soft, anterior, 30% effaced, and 1 cm dilatated. She is experiencing occasional weak contractions throughout the visit. The physician gives her the option of going to the hospital now and being induced, or waiting to go into labor. She decides to wait until the afternoon and then, if no regular contractions start, she will come in for an induction. Four hours later her contractions have started naturally at home. They are coming every three minutes and lasting a full minute when she arrives at the hospital.

Although she had planned to get an epidural early, she is doing very well with the contractions and finds that with the support of the nurse and the Jacuzzi bath, which the nurse encourages her to use, she is getting enough relief that she is considering not getting the epidural. Her labor progresses quickly, and within six hours of being admitted to the hospital she is completely effaced and 9 cm dilatated. The baby is at zero station. Her membranes rupture spontaneously while she is walking back to her bed from the bathroom, and before the nurse can even check the fetal heart tones Margaret cries out, short of breath, and holds her upper abdomen. The nurse gets her back to bed immediately, puts on the call light, and checks her BP and the baby's heart tones. Within a minute her BP drops to 60/40, she becomes faint and then becomes semiconscious, and the fetal heart tone baseline drops to 90 with a prolonged late deceleration. The physician is in the unit and immediately responds. Margaret is rushed to the OR, where a cesarean section is performed and a 6 pound 2 ounce baby boy is delivered. Even with full resuscitative efforts, the APGAR scores are 1 at one minute, 1 at five minutes, and 3 at ten minutes.

Margaret goes into cardiac arrest and is revived. Five minutes after her uterus is sutured from the cesarean section, and her abdomen is being closed, she begins to bleed profusely from every orifice and puncture site. A decision is made to do a hysterectomy while trying to correct her bleeding problem. Margaret has four IVs infusing with blood and expanders under pressure. Once again she is stabilized. An air ambulance is called in, and she is transported by helicopter to the regional high-risk center. Despite the immediate responses from the very beginning by the nursing and medical team, Margaret has another cardiac arrest on board the helicopter and dies. Her baby is also transferred to the high-risk center, and two weeks later he too dies.

Questions

1. Identify three possible causes for her sudden change in condition.

2. Could this problem have been identified prior to the actual crisis?

3. Did Margaret's use of the Jacuzzi tub increase her risk for this complication?

4. What labor factors have been associated with amniotic fluid embolism?

5. List, in order, the immediate nursing actions to be taken when Margaret cried out and within the first three minutes that followed.

6. On autopsy the precipitating problem identified was an amniotic fluid embolism. The immediate response was sudden hypotension, followed by a placenta abruption leading to hemorrhage, shock, and then disseminated intravascular coagulopathy (DIC). Discuss this sequence of events.

7. How frequently do amniotic fluid embolisms occur?

8. What lab tests should the nurse anticipate that the physician will order immediately?

9. List the steps in the neonatal resuscitation.

10. Margaret was being transferred from a small community hospital to a tertiary care center. What is the difference between the levels of maternity care?

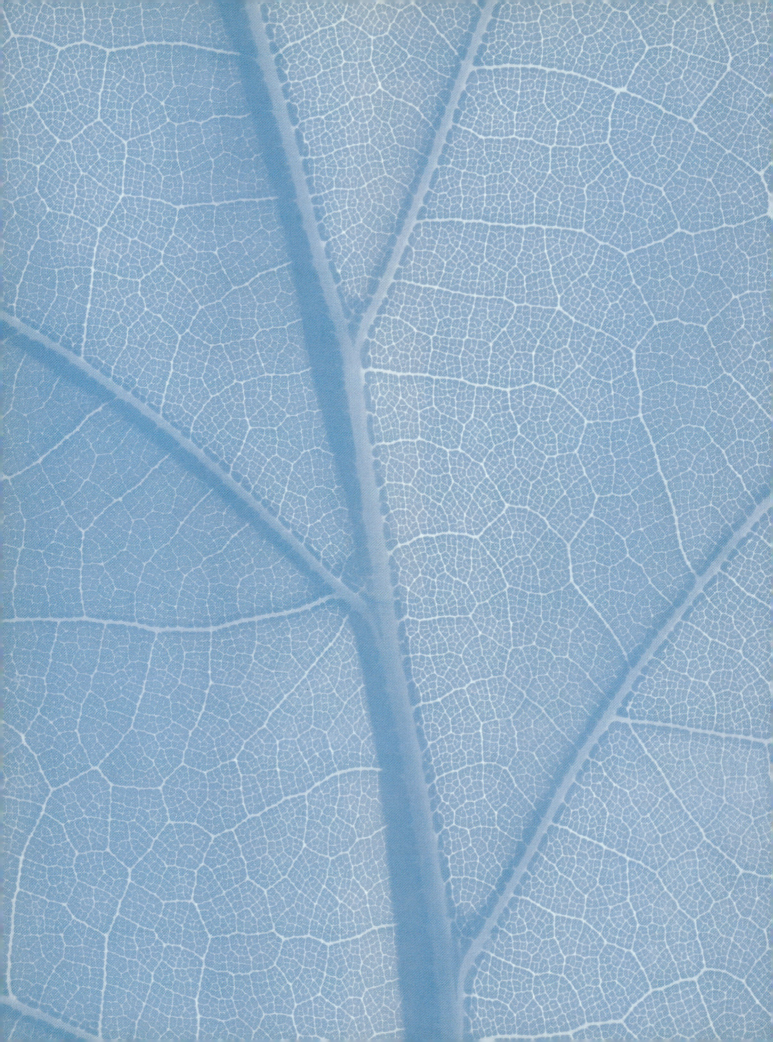

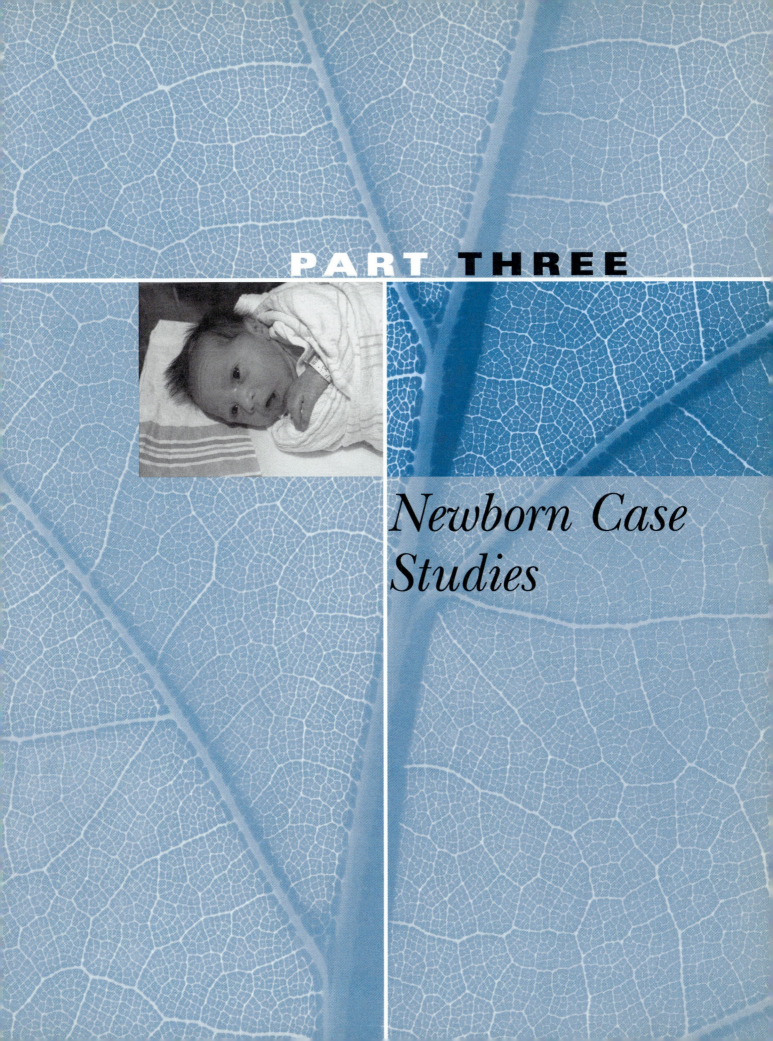

PART THREE

Newborn Case Studies

Baby Nova

AGE

24 hours

SETTING

■ Hospital postpartum unit

CULTURAL CONSIDERATIONS

ETHNICITY

■ White American

PRE-EXISTING CONDITION

CO-EXISTING CONDITION/CURRENT PROBLEM

■ Initiating breastfeeding

COMMUNICATIONS

DISABILITY

SOCIOECONOMIC STATUS

SPIRITUAL/RELIGIOUS

PSYCHOSOCIAL

LEGAL

ETHICAL

PRIORITIZATION

DELEGATION

PHARMACOLOGIC

■ Butorphanol tartrate (Stadol)

ALTERNATIVE THERAPY

SIGNIFICANT HISTORY

■ Delivered by NSVD

NEWBORN

Level of difficulty: Easy

Overview: Requires that the student identify those factors that support and those that interfere with the initiation of breastfeeding. This case gives an example of a common hospital policy that can be detrimental to the mother/infant attachment process. It asks students to be cognizant of policies that may be outdated and are contrary to evidence-based studies. Furthermore, it asks students to consider the responsibility of the nurse in policy making and keeping care practices current with known research.

Client Profile

Baby Nova is 24 hours old. She is full term, weighs 7 pounds 3 ounces, and is 22 inches long. She was born via a NSVD after 12 hours of induced labor. Her mom had butorphanol tartrate (Stadol) for pain relief—last dose two hours prior to birth. After 10 minutes with mom and dad she was taken to the observation nursery until her temperature stabilized. Her APGAR scores were 8 and 9. Admission notes included T 98, HR 110, respirations 44, overall pink, active, and alert. She was given sterile water followed by 5% glucose by a bottle at two hours.

Case Study

The mother received Baby Nova at four hours of age and attempted to breastfeed for the first time. The baby had difficulty taking the nipple and after 30 minutes of trying, the mother, now in tears, called the nurse for help. Upon entering the room the nurse finds the mother in tears, and the baby is sleepy. She states, "She doesn't want the breast. Look, even when I can get her awake she just turns her head away from me." She is attempting to direct the baby's head toward the breast. The baby's maternal grandmother is with her. She is encouraging her daughter to give the baby a bottle since she perceives that her daughter does not have enough milk.

Questions

1. What is the rationale for taking the baby to the nursery for observation after the birth? As a nurse, how can you implement policy changes that reflect current evidence-based practice?

2. Why is Baby Nova given first sterile water and then 5% glucose feedings in the nursery?

3. Why do you think the baby will not feed when her mother offers her the breast?

4. What is happening when the baby looks away from the breast while the mother tries to direct her to the breast?

5. How does the pain medication given the mother affect her attempt to breastfeed at this time?

6. Describe proper positioning at the breast for breastfeeding.

7. Name three things that should have been done differently that would have increased this mother's ability to breastfeed this baby.

8. How can the nurse assist her now?

9. What are the consequences if the baby is given formula now?

10. The mother asks, "How long should I breastfeed?" What is the most appropriate answer?

Baby Haley

AGE

Newborn

SETTING

- Hospital delivery room

CULTURAL CONSIDERATIONS

ETHNICITY

- Black American

PRE-EXISTING CONDITION

CO-EXISTING CONDITION/CURRENT PROBLEM

- Down syndrome

COMMUNICATIONS

DISABILITY

SOCIOECONOMIC STATUS

SPIRITUAL/RELIGIOUS

PSYCHOSOCIAL

- Grieving

LEGAL

ETHICAL

PRIORITIZATION

DELEGATION

PHARMACOLOGIC

ALTERNATIVE THERAPY

SIGNIFICANT HISTORY

- Delivered by NSVD

NEWBORN

Level of difficulty: Easy

Overview: Requires recognition of signs of Down syndrome and critical thinking to assess and plan care for neonate with problems related to congenital anomalies.

Client Profile

Baby Haley's mother is a 26-year-old, G2P1001, MBF. Her first child is a healthy little 6-year-old girl. Mrs. Haley works as a cashier at Wal-Mart. There were no complications identified in the pregnancy, although she did not start prenatal care until her 24th week of pregnancy.

Case Study

Baby Haley has just been born after a two-hour second stage of labor. Immediately at delivery the nurse notes the following:

- Baby Haley lacks tone. He feels like a "bean bag doll."
- His color is dusky.
- He made respiratory effort, but his breathing is irregular and shallow.
- His heart rate is 100 bpm but irregular, with no murmurs.
- When suctioned he reacted by sneezing and gagging.

After resuscitation the nurse continued to examine Baby Haley and further noted:

- He had a large fat pad at the back of his neck.
- He had simian creases on both hands.
- His eyes seemed to be farther apart than usual.
- His ears were low set.
- His tone did not improve after resuscitation even though his color and respirations improved and he was weaned off the oxygen.

Questions

1. What is Baby's Haley's initial APGAR score? List the points for each component.

2. The mother was not screened for congenital anomalies. What might the reason be for this?

3. What congenital defects would the nurse suspect from the observed characteristics?

4. How diagnostic are these observations?

5. If the mother had started prenatal care earlier and had had a triple screen at 18 weeks gestation, what is the possibility that Down syndrome would have been identified?

6. If the triple screen or quad screen had come back positive for Down syndrome, what further testing would have been reommended?

7. List the special observations that the nurse will make on Baby Haley during his transition.

8. The mother wants to nurse her son right after delivery. How should the nurse respond?

9. Baby Haley's mother asks the nurse, "What is wrong with him? My daughter seemed so different at birth." How should the nurse respond?

10. The father walks out of the delivery room, sits in a chair in the hall, and puts his head in his hands and cries. How should the nurse approach him?

Baby Maria

AGE

18 hours

SETTING

- Postpartum unit

CULTURAL CONSIDERATIONS

- Cuban American immigrant traditions

ETHNICITY

- Cuban

PRE-EXISTING CONDITION

CO-EXISTING CONDITION/CURRENT PROBLEM

- Milia; Mongolian spots; acrocyanosis; nipple confusion; formula supplementation

COMMUNICATIONS

DISABILITY

SOCIOECONOMIC STATUS

SPIRITUAL/RELIGIOUS

PSYCHOSOCIAL

- Recent Cuban immigrant

LEGAL

ETHICAL

PRIORITIZATION

DELEGATION

PHARMACOLOGIC

- Meperidine hydrochloride (Demerol)

ALTERNATIVE THERAPY

SIGNIFICANT HISTORY

- Delivered by scheduled cesarean section

NEWBORN

Level of difficulty: Easy

Overview: This case requires that the student identify normal variations in the neonate. Requires identifying those problems created by cesarean section that interfere with breastfeeding and problem solving to reduce these problems.

Client Profile

Baby Maria was born via a repeat cesarean section at 38 weeks gestation in a large teaching hospital. Her mother is a 29-year-old G2P1001, recent Cuban immigrant.

Case Study

Baby Maria has been breastfeeding with formula supplement at night. Her mother is concerned about white spots on her baby's nose and chin and large "bruises" on her buttocks and upper legs. She is also concerned because the baby's feet seem cold and are bluish. Maria's mother asks the nurse to bring her some formula for the baby's afternoon feeding because she does not have enough milk and cannot find a comfortable position for nursing since she is in pain from the cesarean section.

Questions

1. How might the fact that Baby Maria was born by a cesarean section impact her mother's ability to be successful at breastfeeding?

2. What are the implications of Baby Maria being supplemented with formula at night?

3. How should the nurse respond to the mother's request for formula?

4. What suggestion might the nurse give to increase the mother's milk supply?

5. What positions might the nurse assist the mother in that will make her more comfortable for nursing after a cesarean section?

6. Explain the most probable cause of the "white spots on Maria's nose and chin"?

7. How should the nurse explain the "bruises" on the baby's buttocks and legs?

8. What explanation can the nurse give for the condition of the baby's feet?

9. Maria's mom is getting meperidine hydrochloride (Demerol) for pain relief. How can the nurse help Baby Maria's mother to relax and achieve the most effect from her pain medications?

Baby James

AGE

6 hours

SETTING

- Small community hospital nursery

CULTURAL CONSIDERATIONS

ETHNICITY

- Black American

PRE-EXISTING CONDITION

- Fetal tachycardia

CO-EXISTING CONDITION/CURRENT PROBLEM

- Jaundice; low APGARS; hypoglycemia; hypothermia; coarse breath sounds; TTN; RDS

COMMUNICATIONS

DISABILITY

SOCIOECONOMIC STATUS

SPIRITUAL/RELIGIOUS

PSYCHOSOCIAL

LEGAL

ETHICAL

PRIORITIZATION

DELEGATION

PHARMACOLOGIC

ALTERNATIVE THERAPY

SIGNIFICANT HISTORY

- Delivered by NSVD at 36 weeks gestation; no prenatal care; prolonged ruptured membranes

NEWBORN

Level of difficulty: Moderate

Overview: This case requires that the student understand how stress increases the neonate's metabolic rate and the effects this has on the infant's ability to survive. Requires critical thinking regarding differentiating a benign respiratory problem (TTN) and the life threatening condition of RDS. Requires knowledge regarding developing jaundice in the neonate under 24 hours.

Client Profile

Baby James was born via a normal spontaneous vaginal delivery (NSVD) at 36 weeks gestation in a small community hospital. The mother arrived at the emergency room at 9 cm, 100% effaced, reporting ruptured membranes for 22 hours. Baby's fetal heart tones were 170 bpm. The mother delivered in the emergency room 30 minutes after being examined. This is her seventh pregnancy, and she did not have prenatal care.

Case Study

Baby James was admitted to the observation nursery from the emergency room where he was born. He weighed 5 pounds and was 19 inches long. His APGARS were 6 at one minute, and 8 at five minutes. Points were initially taken off for tone, reflexes, and color. His initial glucose was 35 and vital signs were HR 150, respiratory rate 76, temperature 97.2. The nurse noted some nasal flaring, grunting, and coarse breath sounds. He was given 1 ounce of D_5W PO, oxygen therapy; his skin and nasal pharynx were cultured, and he was observed on a warmer with skin probe for temperature monitoring.

At two hours the baby's glucose was 40, the nasal flaring continued, respiratory rate was 100 and irregular with continued coarse breath sounds. He exhibited acrocyanosis, and his temperature was 96.8. The baby was treated for transient tachypnea of the newborn (TTN) with oxygen therapy and a warm environment.

At four hours the nurse noted that the baby was lethargic and difficult to arouse. He appeared pale with circumoral cyanosis, nasal flaring, and grunting with sternal retractions. The nurse notified the pediatrician, an IV was started, and the baby was transferred to the neonatal intensive care unit (NICU) at a hospital in the next town.

At six hours the mother called the NICU to check on his progress and was told that he had subsequently developed jaundice and was on a ventilator.

Questions

1. What is the significance of the fact that this mother had no prenatal care?

2. What are the risks involved in a precipitous delivery?

3. What do you think might have been done differently for this delivery had the mother come in at 4 to 6 cm instead of 9 cm?

4. List the progressive signs of respiratory distress exhibited by this infant after birth.

5. This baby is initially being screened for infection and treated for transient tachypnea of the newborn. What data supports this diagnosis?

6. What is the most likely reason for this baby's initial hypoglycemia?

7. Assess the baby's vital signs. Which ones are within normal range and which ones need attention?

8. List the risk factors that existed for infection.

9. Why is this baby hypothermic, and how does it affect this baby's transition?

10. How significant is the acrocyanosis?

11. What is the significance of jaundice in a 6-hour-old infant?

Baby Ittybit

AGE

48 hours

SETTING

- Home

CULTURAL CONSIDERATIONS

ETHNICITY

- Black American

PRE-EXISTING CONDITION

CO-EXISTING CONDITION/CURRENT PROBLEM

- Physiologic jaundice

COMMUNICATIONS

DISABILITY

SOCIOECONOMIC STATUS

SPIRITUAL/RELIGIOUS

PSYCHOSOCIAL

- Negative familial interference

LEGAL

ETHICAL

PRIORITIZATION

DELEGATION

PHARMACOLOGIC

ALTERNATIVE THERAPY

SIGNIFICANT HISTORY

- Delivered by NSVD

MODERATE

NEWBORN

Level of difficulty: Moderate

Overview: Requires using critical thinking to assess the neonate who is experiencing physiologic jaundice. This case also looks at factors that undermine a mother's confidence in breastfeeding.

Client Profile

Baby Ittybit is a 48-hour-old Black American neonate. He was born at the birth center two days ago. He is breastfeeding well and is active and alert.

Case Study

The nurse is making a home visit to check on the mother and baby. The maternal grandmother is very concerned about the baby since he appears yellow. She had discouraged her daughter from breastfeeding and wanted her to deliver in the hospital. She is convinced that the baby is getting sick due to breastfeeding and being born outside of an acute care facility. The mother is becoming very tearful and losing her confidence.

Questions

1. From an initial assessment, what is the main problem in this situation?

2. What is the most probable explanation for the baby being jaundiced? Give supporting evidence for your answer.

3. Explain the physiology of physiologic jaundice.

4. Baby Ittybit is Black American. How is jaundice assessed in darker skinned infants?

5. Explain how breast milk affects neonatal jaundice.

6. Is it probable that breast milk is the problem? Why or why not?

7. What observations can the nurse make that will help determine if the baby is experiencing pathologic jaundice?

8. List four causes of pathologic jaundice.

9. Describe the four steps of bilirubin metabolism.

10. What are the potential consequences if Baby Ittybit has pathologic jaundice and it is not treated?

11. Outline a teaching plan to educate the parents and grandmother about jaundice and to empower the mother on her ability to make decisions about her baby's care.

Baby Chary

AGE

   24 hours

SETTING

   ■ Newborn nursery

CULTURAL CONSIDERATIONS

ETHNICITY

   ■ White American

PRE-EXISTING CONDITION

CO-EXISTING CONDITION/CURRENT PROBLEM

   ■ Potential hearing loss

COMMUNICATIONS

DISABILITY

SOCIOECONOMIC STATUS

SPIRITUAL/RELIGIOUS

PSYCHOSOCIAL

LEGAL

ETHICAL

PRIORITIZATION

DELEGATION

PHARMACOLOGIC

   ■ Tetracycline; azithromycin (Zithromax); metronidazole (Flagyl); nicotine

ALTERNATIVE THERAPY

SIGNIFICANT HISTORY

   ■ Delivered by NSVD

NEWBORN

Level of difficulty: Moderate

Overview: This case requires that the student understand the connection between maternal prenatal drug ingestion and neonatal hearing. The learner will also be asked to identify various integumentary alterations seen in the newborn.

Client Profile

Baby Chary was born 24 hours ago. Her mother went into labor at 38 weeks gestation and delivered after 16 hours of normal labor and delivery. The pregnancy was essentially normal with the exception that at the beginning of the pregnancy the mother was taking several medications prior to knowing that she was pregnant. The mother was taking a prescription of mocycline hydrochloride (Minocycline) and using topical erythromycin benzoyl peroxide (Benzamycin) gel for some facial acne. She was also taking birth control pills for several months during this period of time in which she was unaware of her pregnancy. The mother smoked a pack of cigarettes a day up to the time she discovered she was pregnant, but then used nicotine gum for a month while she reduced the number of cigarettes she smoked. Finally she was able to quit completely by four months gestation. During her second trimester she developed a severe sinus infection and was treated with prescribed azithromycin (Zithromax), 500 mg times one and then 250 mg a day for four more days. In the third trimester she was prescribed metronidazole (Flagyl) 500 mg bid for 7 days for a Trichomonas vaginitis infection.

Case Study

Baby Chary's APGARS at birth were 7 at one minute and 9 at five minutes, and the baby nursed well right after birth. The nurse notes the following features on an admission physical exam: preauricular skin tag on the right ear, a preauricular sinus on the left ear, and a large pink macular lesion on the back of the neck.

Questions

1. The mother stated that she never missed a birth control pill. What is the possibility of getting pregnant while not missing any pills?

2. What are the risks to the baby since the mother continued to take the birth control pills for the first two months of her pregnancy?

3. The mother asks the nurse what the pink mark is on her baby's neck. The nurse examines the mark and finds that it is small, approximately 1 cm flat with irregular edges. It blanches with pressure, and becomes darker as the baby cries. How should the nurse reply to the mother?

4. The mother notices that the baby does not seem to hear her. When and how will the baby's hearing be checked?

5. Review the medications that the mother took for the acne. What possible consequences do they present for the infant?

6. What is the significance of the skin tag on the baby's right ear?

7. On day three the pediatrician decided to look at the baby's ear canal with an otoscope. Describe how this procedure is done.

8. What are the advantages to early detection of hearing loss?

9. Discuss the mother's illness in the second trimester and her taking the azithromycin (Zithromax) at that time.

10. How does Trichomonas vaginitis affect pregnancy? How safe is metronidazole (Flagyll) in the third trimester?

11. Discuss the mother's use of tobacco and nicotine. Is Baby Chary at increased risk for any health problems because of it?

Baby Cunningham

AGE

3 hours

SETTING

- Hospital

CULTURAL CONSIDERATIONS

ETHNICITY

- White American

PRE-EXISTING CONDITION

- Failed induction

CO-EXISTING CONDITION/CURRENT PROBLEM

- Prematurity; respiratory distress syndrome

COMMUNICATIONS

DISABILITY

SOCIOECONOMIC STATUS

SPIRITUAL/RELIGIOUS

PSYCHOSOCIAL

LEGAL

ETHICAL

PRIORITIZATION

DELEGATION

PHARMACOLOGIC

- Dinoprostone (Cervidil); oxytocin (Pitocin)

ALTERNATIVE THERAPY

SIGNIFICANT HISTORY

- Delivered by cesarean section following labor

NEWBORN

Level of difficulty: Difficult

Overview: Requires critical thinking in order to do gestational age assessment and identify respiratory distress syndrome. Requires identification of the effects of stress on temperature regulation, glucose stores, and respiratory transition.

DIFFICULT

Client Profile

Baby Cunningham was born three hours ago via a cesarean section for a failed induction following a normal pregnancy. The mother had come to the hospital with her membranes intact and having some moderate intermittent Braxton Hicks uterine contractions for the past 24 hours. A vaginal exam revealed a long and thick cervix, which was somewhat anterior and closed. The baby's gestational age was established at 37 weeks by late ultrasound because of an uncertain LMP. Since she was near term and her exam revealed that she was not in active labor, the decision was made to try to induce labor. She was started with a prostaglandin agent dinoprostone (Cervidil), for cervical ripening, then IV oxytocin (Pitocin) to induce and augment labor. She was given an epidural just after the Pitocin was started. Contractions were established at 90 seconds, coming every two minutes. After more than eight hours of labor, her cervix had effaced 60% and only dilated to about 1 cm. The baby developed some repeated prolonged deep late decelerations with poor recovery and minimal short-term variability. Because of the fetal distress, it was decided to turn off the oxytocin (Pitocin) and perform an emergency cesarean section for fetal distress and failure to progress. At delivery the infant was very pale with an extremely slow heart rate, no respiratory effort, and absent tone. Resuscitation included positive pressure ventilation (PPV) by bag and mask with short-term CPR. The baby's APGARS were 3 at one minute, 6 at five minutes, and 8 by ten minutes without any need for epinephrine or sodium bicarbonate. At birth the nurse noticed the following physical characteristics:

- Large amount of lanugo and vernix
- Breasts flat without buds
- Faint plantar creases only
- Equally prominent clitoris and minora
- Slow recoil of ears

The neuromotor exam was not performed due to the persistent depression of the infant's tone and reflexes status post-resuscitation.

Case Study

Baby Cunningham was shown to her parents and transferred to the special care nursery for observation and continued support including oxygen and oxygen saturation monitoring. Under the radiant warmer (Figure 3.1), at 30 minutes of life, the baby was pale and breathing at 88 b/m with some nasal flaring and audible grunting present with some rales heard bilaterally with a stethoscope. Baby Cunningham was continued on blow-by oxygen, warmth, and suctioning prn.

At 45 minutes the respirations were still 88 to 100, with audible grunting, sternal retractions, and nasal flaring. The baby was pale, cyanotic, and dusky even on 100% oxygen by oxyhood with a pulseox saturation of 87%. Her heart rate was 190, and the temperature continued low at 96 in spite of active warming. Random blood glucose was 25 at one hour. The physician ordered an IV to be started with 10% glucose and blood cultures to be done.

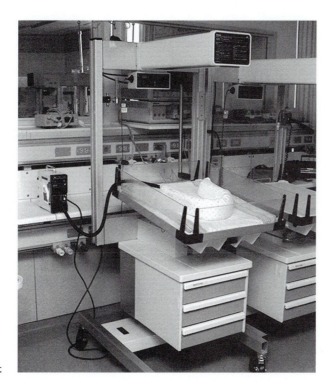

Figure 3.1 *Radiant warmer.*

Questions

1. What is the most likely cause of this infant's distress?

2. List the dangers of elective induction.

3. How accurate are late ultrasounds for establishing gestational age?

4. What is the normal respiratory rate of a neonate at this age? How does Baby Cunningham's compare? Why do you think this is occurring?

5. Assess Baby Cunningham's temperature. Is this normal at this age? Why do you think this is occurring?

6. What is the normal range for neonatal glucose levels? How does Baby Cunningham's compare? Why do you think this is happening, and what problems could arise if it is not corrected?

7. Explain the compensatory principles behind tachypnea, nasal flaring, grunting, and retractions in respiratory distress.

8. How does the environmental temperature affect Baby Cunningham's chances of survival?

9. Why were cultures done?

10. How does the APGAR score differ for the preterm infant as opposed to the full-term one?

11. How might this situation have been avoided?

12. What affects related to parenting can be expected as a result of the birth complications and infant condition?

13. How can the nurse minimize these consequences?

Baby Long

AGE

> 2 hours

SETTING

> ■ Hospital NB nursery

CULTURAL CONSIDERATIONS

ETHNICITY

> ■ White American

PRE-EXISTING CONDITION

CO-EXISTING CONDITION/CURRENT PROBLEM

> ■ Thrombocytopenia

COMMUNICATIONS

DISABILITY

SOCIOECONOMIC STATUS

SPIRITUAL/RELIGIOUS

PSYCHOSOCIAL

LEGAL

ETHICAL

PRIORITIZATION

DELEGATION

PHARMACOLOGIC

ALTERNATIVE THERAPY

SIGNIFICANT HISTORY

> ■ Cesarean section

NEWBORN

Level of difficulty: Difficult

Overview: The case examines the relationship of placenta abruption and development of thrombocytopenia in the newborn. The learner is asked to identify risk factors for and signs and symptoms in the neonate, identify risks associated with thrombocytopenia, and plan the care for the infant.

DIFFICULT

Client Profile

Baby Long was delivered by an emergency cesarean section two hours ago because of some fetal tachycardia and maternal fever of 101.8. The pregnancy was complicated by preterm premature rupture of membranes (PPROM), which occurred following an automobile accident two days ago at which time the mother sustained some minor trauma to the abdomen. During the delivery it was noted that she had developed a small to moderate placenta abruption. The baby's gestational age was determined to be about 32 weeks. The mother later developed disseminated intravascular coagulopathy (DIC) and is currently in critical condition in the Intensive Care Unit.

Case Study

The baby required full resuscitation at birth and had APGARS of 4 and 5 at one and five minutes. The ten minute APGAR was 6. She was immediately admitted to the NICU on a ventilator.

Questions

1. During the initial exam the nurse notes that the baby had petechiae on his abdomen and face and also notes that there is some oozing of blood from the venipuncture sites. List possible causes of this finding.

2. The nurse puts a call in to the physician. What initial laboratory studies should the nurse anticipate?

3. How might results be affected if the nurse decides to collect the blood for these tests by a heel stick?

4. The baby's platelet count is 60,000 units per liter. Assess this finding.

5. What would be the next anticipated set of lab tests that might be needed?

6. Would the nurse anticipate a spinal tap to be a part of the sepsis workup?

7. Should the nurse anticipate the insertion of an umbilical arterial catheter?

8. What other signs might the nurse note that would be associated with thrombocytopenia?

9. Baby Long was also diagnosed with intraventricular hemorrhage (IVH). What factors contributed directly to this condition?

10. List all of possible etiologies that are present in the delivery history.

11. What further lab tests might be included in the evaluation of this thrombocytopenia?

12. What is the treatment that the nurse should anticipate for this infant's thrombocytopenia?

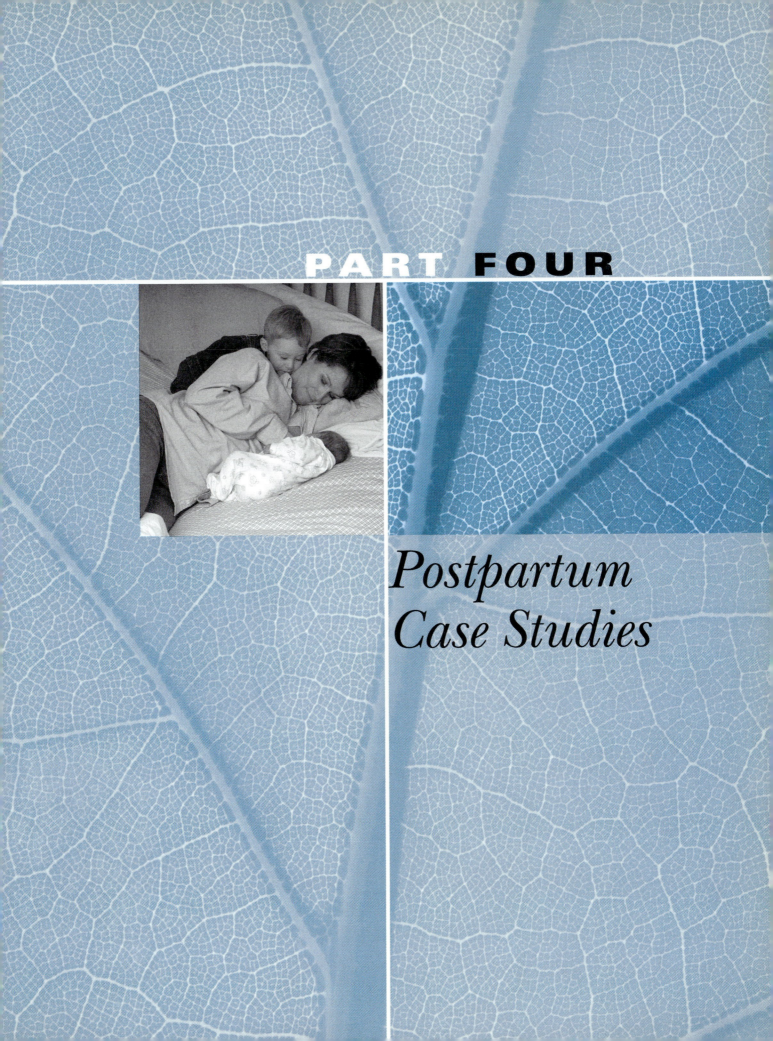

PART FOUR

*Postpartum
Case Studies*

Molly

AGE

29

SETTING

■ Hospital postpartum unit

CULTURAL CONSIDERATIONS

■ White American culture

ETHNICITY

■ White American

PRE-EXISTING CONDITION

CO-EXISTING CONDITION/CURRENT PROBLEM

■ PP blues; 4th-degree laceration;
postpartum hemorrhage

COMMUNICATIONS

DISABILITY

SOCIOECONOMIC STATUS

SPIRITUAL/RELIGIOUS

PSYCHOSOCIAL

■ Previous positive home birth experience

LEGAL

ETHICAL

PRIORITIZATION

DELEGATION

PHARMACOLOGIC

ALTERNATIVE THERAPY

SIGNIFICANT HISTORY

■ Multipara

POSTPARTUM

Level of difficulty: Easy

Overview: Requires using critical thinking to assess and plan care for a woman experiencing postpartum blues following a postpartum hemorrhage and a fourth-degree laceration.

Client Profile

Molly is a 29-year-old, G2P2002, MWF. She is breastfeeding. Her first baby is two years old, and she breastfed that baby for one year. Her first baby weighed 8 pounds and was born at home, and she felt that it had been a wonderful experience. She delivered in the squatting position over an intact perineum, walked and danced throughout her labor, and used her bath to relax through much of the first stage. She had recently moved and could not find a midwife to help her with a home birth this time.

This delivery was induced at 40 weeks 2 days with Pitocin. After 6 hours she had an epidural for anesthesia. The baby was born vaginally with forceps. The baby weighed 7 pounds 2 ounces. She experienced a fourth-degree laceration following a mediolateral episiotomy. Her estimated blood loss (EBL) was 1000 mL.

Case Study

At 24 hours postpartum, Molly is feeling depressed. The nurse finds her crying quietly while breastfeeding her baby. The baby is feeding well. Molly's older baby is tucked in the bed next to her, asleep.

Questions

1. Make a list of possible reasons for Molly's tears.

2. What is the relationship between episiotomy and third- and fourth-degree lacerations?

3. What are the rationales for induction?

4. Molly had already experienced a natural birth and was satisfied with her birth. What factors may have caused her to ask for an epidural this time?

5. What pelvic structures are involved in a fourth-degree laceration?

6. What special precautions are needed for the woman who has a fourth-degree laceration?

7. What is the normal amount of blood loss for a vaginal birth?

8. How does Molly's loss compare?

9. List at least two complications that may occur as a result of her postpartum hemorrhage.

10. How should the nurse best approach Molly at this time?

11. If Molly's older baby wishes to resume breastfeeding, what should she do?

CASE STUDY 2

Candace

AGE

23

SETTING

■ Home

CULTURAL CONSIDERATIONS

ETHNICITY

■ White American

PRE-EXISTING CONDITION

CO-EXISTING CONDITION/CURRENT PROBLEM

■ Blocked duct; mastitis; postpartum blues

COMMUNICATIONS

DISABILITY

SOCIOECONOMIC STATUS

SPIRITUAL/RELIGIOUS

PSYCHOSOCIAL

LEGAL

ETHICAL

PRIORITIZATION

DELEGATION

PHARMACOLOGIC

■ Ampicillin

ALTERNATIVE THERAPY

SIGNIFICANT HISTORY

■ Primipara

POSTPARTUM

Level of difficulty: Easy

Overview: Requires using critical thinking to assess and provide care for a woman with mastitis.

Client Profile

Candace is a 23-year-old, G1P1, MWF who delivered a 7 pound 8 ounce baby boy three weeks ago at the local birth center. She is very happy about her birth and is adjusting well to motherhood. She breastfed her baby a few minutes after the birth and has continued to exclusively breastfeed him. She intends to breastfeed for at least a year, probably starting him on solid foods around six months. Prior to the pregnancy Candace was a busy office executive in a local shipping firm. She is on a six-week leave of absence. She plans to pump her breast milk for the baby when she returns to work. She is hoping that her mother-in-law, who will be caring for the baby, will be able to bring the baby to her workplace at least once a day, at noon, to breastfeed and then give the baby the breast milk she has left from a bottle for the other feedings. Her mother-in-law will be arriving from out of state in two weeks. Candace is a very "in control person." She plans everything in her life, and up to this point the world has respected her wishes.

Case Study

Candace called the birth center this morning crying. Her breast on the left side is so sore she cannot stand to have the baby nurse on that side, and to make matters worse, that is the only side the baby will take. For the last 12 hours the baby seems to want to nurse all the time or just cries and sucks his fist. She feels sick, cannot get anything done at home, and at 2 p.m. is still in her pajamas with last night's dinner and this morning's breakfast dishes still in the sink. She and her husband had an argument this morning and he left for work angry and overtired after getting no sleep all night from the baby crying. He just wants her to stop being so stubborn, since she obviously doesn't have enough milk, and give the baby some formula. Her car has broken down and she has no other source of transportation. The nurse working at the birth center offers to make a home visit.

Questions

1. Prior to arriving at the home, what problems does the nurse anticipate at this visit?

2. Make a list of the questions that the nurse will ask Candace at the home visit.

3. Make a list of the observations that need to be made at the home visit.

4. Explain the process of supply and demand as it applies to breastfeeding and milk supply.

5. Why does it appear to Candace's husband that Candace has lost her milk?

6. On arrival the nurse finds that Candace's left breast nipple is cracked and bleeding slightly. The nurse also notes that Candace has a fever of 101.2°, seems lethargic, and has an area about the size of a quarter on the underside of her right breast that is firm, red, and warm. Candace tells the nurse that she feels like she has the flu. What is Candace's problem, what probably caused it, and what is the nurse's next action?

7. The CNM at the birth center calls in a prescription for ampicillin 500 mg po qid for 10 days. Candace starts crying and asks if this means she can no longer breastfeed. What is the nurse's best response?

8. Outline a teaching plan to reduce the possibility of Candace having another mastitis infection.

9. Why did the baby only want to nurse on the left side?

10. How can the nurse help Candace get him to also nurse on the right side?

11. Where can the nurse refer Candace for support with her breastfeeding?

12. Candace plans to return to work in two weeks. Make a list of decisions and possible problems that she will have to work through during these next two weeks, and after she returns to work, to prepare her and the baby for this transition. Provide alternative suggestions for her to consider.

CASE STUDY 3

Juanita

AGE

24

SETTING

■ Home

CULTURAL CONSIDERATIONS

■ Cuban traditions

ETHNICITY

■ Cuban American

PRE-EXISTING CONDITION

CO-EXISTING CONDITION/CURRENT PROBLEM

■ Rh negative

COMMUNICATIONS

DISABILITY

SOCIOECONOMIC STATUS

SPIRITUAL/RELIGIOUS

PSYCHOSOCIAL

■ Cultural conflicts

LEGAL

ETHICAL

PRIORITIZATION

DELEGATION

PHARMACOLOGIC

■ Rh_o(D) immune globulin (human) (RhoGAM)

ALTERNATIVE THERAPY

SIGNIFICANT HISTORY

■ Primipara

POSTPARTUM

Level of difficulty: Easy

Overview: This case looks at some beliefs common in the Cuban culture, problems that arise from culture conflict between a mother-in-law and the husband, and differences between the daughter and her mother on expectations for postpartum. It also looks at the effects of emotional stress on the breast-feeding process.

Client Profile

Juanita is a 24-year-old, MHF. She is a gravida 1 para 1. Juanita emigrated from Cuba to Miami, Florida several years ago. She has a college education and has read everything she can get her hands on about pregnancy, infant care, and breastfeeding. Her mother just arrived from Cuba two days ago to stay with Juanita and her husband and to help care for her new grandchild. Juanita gave birth three days ago at the local community hospital. She and her husband are very happy about their new daughter. Juanita was discharged from the hospital with the baby yesterday. This morning she called the hospital saying that she was experiencing terrible constipation and was having problems breastfeeding. She asked for a nurse to come to her home for a home visit to help her.

Case Study

When the nurse arrives Juanita is alone with the baby. Her husband went grocery shopping and her mother has gone to the Laundromat^SM to do the washing. Juanita seems happy to see the nurse. They talk for a while and then Juanita bursts into tears. She explains to the nurse that her mother and her husband have been at odds since she got home from the hospital. Her husband is an American and wants very much to be involved in his baby's care, but her mother is from Cuba and sees baby care as her role, and only her role. She even tends to push Juanita aside when it comes to baby care. She also states that she finds many of her mother's ideas old-fashioned, and this is driving her crazy. They all live in a two-bedroom home and the tension is causing problems between Juanita and her husband. "I love my husband, but I can't hurt my mom. I just don't know what to do."

Questions

1. How might the tension between Juanita's mother and husband, and between Juanita and her mother, be affecting Juanita's breastfeeding?

2. How might the problem have been avoided?

3. What suggestions might the nurse give Juanita to relieve the constipation?

4. How will the nurse assess her breastfeeding problems?

5. Are there any community resources that might be helpful for this family?

6. Two days after her delivery, Juanita was given a shot of RhoGAM. At this home visit she asks the nurse why she needed it and if she would have problems with her next pregnancy. How should the nurse reply?

7. Juanita would like to attend a new mothers' group that meets in two weeks. Her mother said that she should not go out for at least 30 days. Juanita is unhappy about this and asks the nurse if she can go. How should the nurse reply?

8. The nurse does an exam on the infant and notices a safety pin on the baby's undershirt with a religious medal on it. What is the significance of this finding?

9. The baby also has a piece of string in the shape of a circle stuck to her forehead. Juanita looks embarrassed when she sees that the nurse notices the string. What is the significance of the string?

10. Juanita tells the nurse that she would like to take a shower and wants to know if it is okay. How should the nurse respond?

Daphne

AGE

14

SETTING

■ Clinic

CULTURAL CONSIDERATIONS

ETHNICITY

■ White American

PRE-EXISTING CONDITION

CO-EXISTING CONDITION/CURRENT PROBLEM

■ Thyrotoxicosis; BF problems; depression; weight loss; fatigue; palpitations; memory loss; swollen cervical glands

COMMUNICATIONS

DISABILITY

SOCIOECONOMIC STATUS

SPIRITUAL/RELIGIOUS

PSYCHOSOCIAL

■ Depression

LEGAL

ETHICAL

PRIORITIZATION

DELEGATION

PHARMACOLOGIC

ALTERNATIVE THERAPY

SIGNIFICANT HISTORY

■ Primipara

MODERATE

POSTPARTUM

Level of difficulty: Moderate

Overview: Requires assessing a postpartum woman at three weeks after delivery to rule out thyroid disease.

Client Profile

Daphne is a 14-year-old, SWF, G1P1 who delivered three weeks ago. She is bottle-feeding at this time. Although she had intended to breastfeed, she stopped after two weeks due to sore nipples and concerns about not having enough breast milk.

Case Study

Her mother calls the clinic to report that Daphne seems very moody, depressed, and agitated. She has lost over 10 pounds in one week despite an increased appetite; she complains of headaches, fatigue, palpitations, memory loss, and swollen glands in her neck.

Questions

1. Identify at least three questions the nurse should ask Daphne's mother during this initial phone call.

2. Give three possible explanations for Daphne's symptoms.

3. The nurse tells Daphne's mother to bring her to the clinic for evaluation. The CNM orders a TSH. Why?

4. Which of Daphne's symptoms can be associated with thyroid disease?

5. Her results for her thyroid stimulating hormone (TSH) are 0.24 μIU/mL What is the most probable diagnosis?

6. What additional test will probably be ordered?

7. What are the possible consequences if hyperthyroidism is the problem and it is not diagnosed?

8. Describe the normal involution to be expected for Daphne at this time.

9. What are the most common reasons women decide not to breastfeed after they have started?

10. Daphne states that she is very disappointed that she is not breastfeeding and would like to try to start to breastfeed again. She has bottle-fed for one week now. What is the best response by the nurse?

Sueata

AGE	**SPIRITUAL/RELIGIOUS**
26	
SETTING	**PSYCHOSOCIAL**
■ Hospital postpartum unit	■ No support from fob
CULTURAL CONSIDERATIONS	**LEGAL**
■ Pakistani traditions	
ETHNICITY	**ETHICAL**
■ Pakistani	
PRE-EXISTING CONDITION	**PRIORITIZATION**
CO-EXISTING CONDITION/CURRENT PROBLEM	**DELEGATION**
COMMUNICATIONS	**PHARMACOLOGIC**
DISABILITY	**ALTERNATIVE THERAPY**
SOCIOECONOMIC STATUS	**SIGNIFICANT HISTORY**
■ Student	■ Primigravida

MODERATE

POSTPARTUM

Level of difficulty: Moderate

Overview: Requires an understanding of the Pakistani culture and the low status of women in that culture.

Client Profile

Sueata has been in the United States for four years. She is from a wealthy family in Pakistan. She is on a student visa, which expires in two months. She fell in love with an American student, and he is the father of her baby. They had an argument when she was seven months pregnant, and he has not called her since. She is 26 years old and this was her first pregnancy. The baby is a girl. Sueata is bottle-feeding.

Case Study

Sueata is two days postpartum. She is scheduled for discharge in the morning. The nurse finds her crying quietly, holding her baby in her arms.

Questions

1. The nurse begins to go over discharge instructions with Sueata. Make a list of the routine discharge instructions given to women who have had normal spontaneous vaginal deliveries.

2. Sueata pushes her baby away and cries out, "I hate you. Why couldn't you have been a boy?" How should the nurse respond?

3. Sueata asks about adoption. This is the first time that she has even mentioned that she was thinking about giving her baby up for adoption. How should the nurse approach this subject?

4. Sueata hands the nurse a letter from the immigration service stating that her student visa will expire in two months. Sueata explains through her tears that if she goes home she will be killed. She has dishonored her family by getting preg-

nant, and they do not want her back. If she goes home, they may even hire someone to kill her. How likely is it that this story may be true? Discuss the status of women in the Pakastani culture.

5. What resources might the nurse offer Sueata?

6. How is childbearing viewed in the Pakastani culture?

7. Will the baby have United States or Pakistani citizenship?

8. What methods of birth control might be acceptable to Sueata?

9. What specific instructions does she need to care for her breasts since she is not breastfeeding?

10. Outline information on formula preparation.

Roquanda

AGE

24

SETTING

- Hospital postpartum unit

CULTURAL CONSIDERATIONS

- Jamician Rastafarian culture

ETHNICITY

- Black American

PRE-EXISTING CONDITION

- ML episiotomy; vacuum extractor; Pitocin-augmented labor and birth; epidural anesthesia

CO-EXISTING CONDITION/CURRENT PROBLEM

- PP hemorrhage

COMMUNICATIONS

DISABILITY

SOCIOECONOMIC STATUS

SPIRITUAL/RELIGIOUS

- Rastafarian

PSYCHOSOCIAL

LEGAL

ETHICAL

PRIORITIZATION

DELEGATION

PHARMACOLOGIC

- Hemabate; Pitocin; Methergine

ALTERNATIVE THERAPY

SIGNIFICANT HISTORY

- Multipara

POSTPARTUM

Level of difficulty: Difficult

Overview: Requires critical thinking to assess, determine cause, and treat a client who experiences postpartum hemorrhage.

DIFFICULT

Client Profile   **Roquanda** is a 24-year-old, G4P3003, MBF. Her oldest child is 3½ years old. She delivered a 9 pound 12 ounce baby boy following an 18-hour Pitocin-augmented labor with epidural anesthesia this morning. Her second stage was two hours. She was given a mediolateral episiotomy, and the baby's head was delivered by vacuum extractor after she experienced difficulty pushing. Her estimated blood loss (EBL) was 400 mL right after delivery. Immediately after delivery her VS were BP 110/70, temperature 98, pulse 68, and respirations 20. She plans to bottle-feed.

Case Study   Roquanda delivered two hours ago and has just been transferred to the postpartum floor with an IV of lactated ringers, which is to be discontinued when it is finished. Upon assessing her, the postpartum nurse notes that Roquanda is trickling blood from the vagina and has soaked a pad about 30 to 40 minutes after she changes it. Her vital signs are BP 90/68, pulse 100, and respiration 28. She appears restless.

Questions

1. Name three common sources of postpartum hemorrhage. Compare and contrast them according to the signs and symptoms, precipitating factors, and treatment for each.

2. What is the normal expected blood loss for a vaginal delivery?

3. Was Roquanda's blood loss normal?

4. What factors increase the initial blood loss in delivery?

5. List four history factors that increase Roquanda's risk for postpartum hemorrhage.

6. List four labor and delivery factors that increased her risk.

7. Assess her vital signs. Are these normal for postpartum?

8. If not, what is the significance of them?

9. List at least six other signs of shock related to hypovolemia.

10. List at least two consequences of postpartum hemorrhage.

11. Why is Roquanda at an even higher risk for problems related to postpartum hemorrhage?

12. When would you expect Roquanda's hematocrit to be checked? If she had a postpartum hemorrhage, how would you expect it to be reflected in the hematocrit?

13. Roquanda's hematocrit is low, and the certified nurse midwife prescribes iron supplements. The nurse is discharging her on her third postpartum day. What information about taking iron supplements needs to be included in teaching Roquanda?

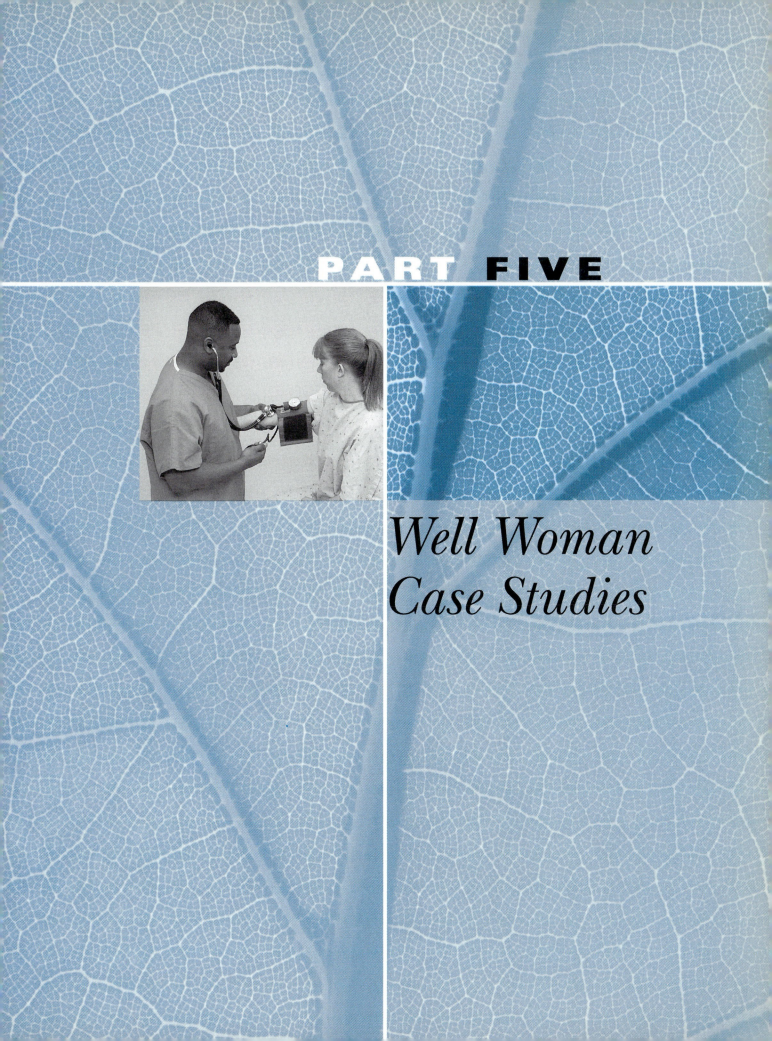

PART FIVE

Well Woman
Case Studies

Carina

AGE

15

SETTING

■ Certified Nurse Midwife's office

CULTURAL CONSIDERATIONS

ETHNICITY

■ White American

PRE-EXISTING CONDITION

■ Anorexia

CO-EXISTING CONDITION/CURRENT PROBLEM

■ Primary amenorrhea

COMMUNICATIONS

DISABILITY

SOCIOECONOMIC STATUS

SPIRITUAL/RELIGIOUS

■ Baptist

PSYCHOSOCIAL

■ Suspected abuse

LEGAL

■ Minor

ETHICAL

■ Self-determination vs rights of parent

PRIORITIZATION

DELEGATION

PHARMACOLOGIC

ALTERNATIVE THERAPY

SIGNIFICANT HISTORY

WELL WOMAN

Level of difficulty: Easy

Overview: Requires using critical thinking to assess teen for primary amenorrhea. Requires skills in assessing communications with teen regarding sexuality and related risks.

Client Profile   **Carina** is a 15-year-old, SWF who has been brought to the midwife's office by her mother. She is five feet five inches, and her current weight is 103 pounds. Her mother states that she is not sexually active.

Case Study   Carina's mother expresses concern that Carina has not yet started her menstrual periods. The nurse is taking an initial history and preparing her for the CNM to do her physical exam. Carina indicates that she does not want her mother present for the history and physical. There does not seem to be tension between them, but Carina indicates that she is old enough to be seen alone. Her mother agrees and returns to the waiting room. During the interview Carina is adamant that she is not sexually active. However, after a period of time she does admit to the nurse that she does engage in casual oral sex because it makes her popular. Besides, she does not consider that having sex. She states that she sees nothing wrong with oral sex but would never have intercourse because, "I am not that kind of girl." During the physical exam, the midwife notes that the inner aspects of Carina's arms are bruised and there is an unusual mark on her breast that could be a bite mark. When Carina is questioned about this, she flippantly states that "Oh, that's my boyfriend. He gets a little carried away sometimes."

Questions

1. Since Carina is a minor and does require her mother's consent to have health care, is it necessary for her mother to be present during the history and physical?

2. How does Carina's description of her sexual activity impact the manner in which the nurse will pursue the interview?

3. Does Carina need a PAP smear and/or STI testing?

4. What particular observations will be important for the nurse and the CNM to help determine the cause of her amenorrhea?

5. List five factors that may contribute to the fact that Carina has not yet started her periods.

6. What possible psychosocial impact might this situation have on Carina?

7. Develop a plan for addressing the abuse situation.

8. List four questions specifically intended to explore possible abuse that would be appropriate at this visit.

9. Outline a teaching plan for Carina.

10. Should Carina be offered birth control?

Cyndie

AGE	**SPIRITUAL/RELIGIOUS**
28	
SETTING	**PSYCHOSOCIAL**
■ Women's clinic	
CULTURAL CONSIDERATIONS	**LEGAL**
ETHNICITY	**ETHICAL**
■ Black American	
PRE-EXISTING CONDITION	**PRIORITIZATION**
CO-EXISTING CONDITION/CURRENT PROBLEM	**DELEGATION**
■ Pelvic inflammatory disease (PID); gonorrhea; chlamydia	
COMMUNICATIONS	**PHARMACOLOGIC**
DISABILITY	**ALTERNATIVE THERAPY**
	SIGNIFICANT HISTORY
SOCIOECONOMIC STATUS	■ Primipara

WELL WOMAN

Level of Difficulty: Moderate

Overview: This case requires that the student use critical thinking to assess and provide care for a client with PID.

Client Profile

Cyndie is a 28-year-old, G1P1, MBF. Her first child is six years old. She and her husband have been trying, without success, to conceive for the past four years. Her first pregnancy was completely normal, and the baby was delivered via a normal spontaneous vaginal delivery at a birth center. Cyndie works as a television announcer.

Case Study

Cyndie is being seen today at the Women's clinic with a vaginal discharge, pelvic pain, and a fever of 101.6°F. A pregnancy test is negative. She has a purulent, irritating vaginal discharge, feels nauseated all the time, and has dysuria.

Questions

1. What test should the nurse anticipate?

2. The client is diagnosed with gonorrhea. What other infection is commonly found with gonorrhea?

3. Just after her last baby was born Cyndie was diagnosed with gonorrhea/chlamydia infections and treated. How might these infections leave her with secondary infertility?

4. Cyndie does not have any drug allergies. What is the most common treatment for these infections?

5. Should she be re-screened? If so, when?

6. Is the clinician required to report these diseases to the public health department? If yes, how is this done?

7. Cyndie also complains of pain around the opening of her vagina on the right side. On inspection the clinician finds an enlarged glandular lump around 2 cm in diameter. This is most probably what?

8. Cyndie also jumps when the clinician moves her cervix. What conditions is cervical motion tenderness (Chandelier's sign) associated with?

9. Outline the teaching the nurse needs to provide to Cyndie prior to her leaving the office today.

10. If Cyndie were pregnant, how would her treatment be different?

Anna

AGE

36

SETTING

- Well Woman clinic

CULTURAL CONSIDERATIONS

ETHNICITY

- Black American

PRE-EXISTING CONDITION

CO-EXISTING CONDITION/CURRENT PROBLEM

- Breast lump; fatigue

COMMUNICATIONS

DISABILITY

SOCIOECONOMIC STATUS

SPIRITUAL/RELIGIOUS

PSYCHOSOCIAL

LEGAL

ETHICAL

PRIORITIZATION

DELEGATION

PHARMACOLOGIC

- Oral contraceptive pills (OCP)

ALTERNATIVE THERAPY

SIGNIFICANT HISTORY

- Multipara

WELL WOMAN

Level of difficulty: Moderate

Overview: Requires critical thinking to differentiate signs associated with benign breast disease from those associated with serious breast lumps.

Client Profile

Anna is a 36-year-old, G4P4, MBF. Anna just moved to Miami three months ago. She is using OCPs for contraception. She has a 10-year-old son and three daughters ages 9, 7, and 4. She breastfed all of her children for at least a year. She is active in all of her children's activities. She is a baseball coach, helps at the junior high in the book store, is on the PTSA (parent teacher student association) planning committee, and keeps the books for her husband's business. Lately she has been feeling more tired than usual.

Case Study

Anna is being seen at the Well Woman clinic for her annual exam. She is actually six months overdue, but last week when doing a breast self-exam she noticed a small lump in her right breast. There were no dimpling or retractions noted on the breast.

Questions

1. What is the significance of the fact that Anna breastfed all of her children for at least a year each?

2. What screening and diagnostic tests are appropriate for Anna at this visit?

3. Anna describes the lump as very small, having irregular edges and not painful. Any clinically palpable mass requires further assessment. What type of lump commonly presents with these characteristics?

4. The nurse examines Anna and finds the lump is fixed and located in the outer upper quadrant of the breast. Are these additional findings reassuring or non-reassuring?

5. The nurse also notices no scaling or nipple discharge and no infraclavicular or supraclavicular adenopathy. However, she did note edema in the auxiliary area of Anna's right arm. What is the significance of this?

6. Which screening test for breast cancer is most appropriate to start with for Anna—an ultrasound or a mammogram?

7. If the mammogram reveals a suspicious lump, what will be the next step to diagnosis if it is cancer?

8. Give at least two possible causes of Anna's fatigue that are not related to the breast lump.

9. List at least three questions that the nurse needs to ask Anna to help determine the cause of her fatigue.

10. Identify two community resources that can offer support to Anna and her family if the breast lump is cancerous.

11. Are Black women more or less at risk for breast cancer?

Jodi

AGE

31

SETTING

■ Certified Nurse Midwife's office

CULTURAL CONSIDERATIONS

ETHNICITY

■ Hispanic American

PRE-EXISTING CONDITION

CO-EXISTING CONDITION/CURRENT PROBLEM

■ Abnormal PAP; condylomata acuminata human papillomavirus; gonorrhea; chlamydia

COMMUNICATIONS

DISABILITY

SOCIOECONOMIC STATUS

SPIRITUAL/RELIGIOUS

PSYCHOSOCIAL

LEGAL

ETHICAL

PRIORITIZATION

DELEGATION

PHARMACOLOGIC

■ Flagyl; 2.5% Nupercainal ointment; doxycycline; erythromycin; azithromycin; ofloxicin; ceftriaxone; cefotaxime; spectinomycin; ciprofloxacin; alendronate (Fosamax); raloxifen (Evista)

■ HRT therapy; Depo-Provera; clonidine; trichloroacetic acid (TCA); podophyllin; 5-FU or imiquimod cream

ALTERNATIVE THERAPY

■ Black cohosh

SIGNIFICANT HISTORY

■ Multipara

MODERATE

WELL WOMAN

Level of difficulty: Moderate

Overview: Requires the student to use critical thinking to assess a client who has an abnormal PAP and to provide education for that client.

Client Profile

Jodi is a 31-year-old G2P2, MHF. She works full time as a high school algebra teacher. Her two children are 7 and 8 years old. She is five feet three inches, and her weight is 112 pounds. She does not want any more children and her current birth control is the contraceptive patch.

Family History: Both of Jodi's parents are alive and well. She has two sisters who are also alive and well. Her maternal grandfather died of a heart attack at age 62. Her other grandparents are all still alive and well.

Medical/Surgical History: Benign

OB/GYN History: She has had two full term normal spontaneous deliveries. Both babies were healthy and appropriately grown (AGA). Prior to her first baby she had a routine PAP smear that was ASCUS with atypia favoring inflammation. This was determined to be bacterial vaginosis, and she was treated with Flagyl. Her next two PAP smears after that were normal. Then during her second pregnancy, she had a routine PAP smear done, which showed ASCUS with atypia now favoring HPV infection. Acetic acid 5% was swabbed on the cervix and several small areas turned white. She was asymptomatic and there were no changes in the lesions throughout the pregnancy. After delivery she returned for a normal postpartum visit and another repeat PAP smear, which again showed ASCUS with atypia favoring HPV; she was sent for a colposcopy and was successfully treated with cryotherapy with complete resolution. After the cryotherapy her repeat PAP smears were all normal. She was told that no more follow-up would be needed since her PAP smears have all been normal since.

Case Study

It has been seven years since her abnormal PAPs. Jodi is now being seen in the office today for her annual exam and a routine repeat PAP test. During the exam the CNM noticed a small external venereal wart present on the inner surface of the labia. A vaginal cervical exam revealed some slight acteowhite cervical changes present. A PAP smear and DNA probe for gonorrhea and chlamydia were done. Local treatment was started with topical podophyllin solution to the wart.

The current repeat PAP smear came back showing high-grade sqamous interepithelial lesion (HGSIL) with high-grade SIL changes. She was sent for a colposcopy, and the biopsy showed severe cervical dysplasia favoring carcinoma in situ. The DNA probe was positive for both gonorrhea and chlamydia, and she was treated. The CNM tried to do some patient counseling with Jodi, but she was totally distraught and was angrily going to confront her husband, who denied having any affairs. She told the CNM that she has been totally faithful to her husband and does not understand how she could have gotten these diseases. She asks if it is possible that she got them at the high school swimming pool where she has been taking her children to swim on the weekends.

Questions

1. Discuss HPV infections.

2. If a client complains of discomfort associated with the HPV treatment, what suggestions can the nurse give her for pain relief?

3. How should the nurse respond to Jodi's question about the swimming pool?

4. Since this last PAP came back showing high-grade SIL changes, what treatment should the nurse anticipate that Jodi will be referred for?

5. What is the significance of the different grades of different PAP smear abnormalities?

6. What is the significance of and treatment for gonorrhea and chlamydia?

7. Jodi says she is tired of using birth control and asks the nurse about permanent sterilization. How should the nurse reply?

8. What are the clinical consequences of a premature surgical hysterectomy?

9. What are the different treatment options available for these types of cutaneous lesion?

10. What type of continuing patient instructions and follow-up will be needed?

11. Will the partner need to be treated for any of the infections?

Jing

AGE

36

SETTING

- Infertility specialty center

CULTURAL CONSIDERATIONS

- Shinto health beliefs

ETHNICITY

- Asian American

PRE-EXISTING CONDITION

- Dysmenorrhea; dyspareunia; increasingly irregular menses; chronic pelvic pain

CO-EXISTING CONDITION/CURRENT PROBLEM

- Endometriosis; infertility; strangulated right ovary

COMMUNICATIONS

DISABILITY

SOCIOECONOMIC STATUS

- IVF is very expensive

SPIRITUAL/RELIGIOUS

- IVF procedures/options; Shinto

PSYCHOSOCIAL

- Stress secondary to reproductive disturbance

LEGAL

ETHICAL

- Destruction of embryo vs ability to carry to viability

PRIORITIZATION

DELEGATION

PHARMACOLOGIC

- Clomiphene citrate (Clomid); Lupron; Synarel

ALTERNATIVE THERAPY

- Accupuncture

SIGNIFICANT HISTORY

- Nulligravida; dysmenorrhea; dyspareunia; increasing irregular menses; chronic pelvic pain

MODERATE

WELL WOMAN

Level of difficulty: Moderate

Overview: Requires understanding endometriosis and its effects on fertility and Shinto health belief system.

Client Profile

Jing is a 36-year-old, G0, married, Asian female who has been previously seen in the clinic for an infertility workup and treatment. She has been having unprotected sexual intercourse for the past 24 months without any conception to date. Her gynecological history includes a history of dysmenorrhea, dyspareunia, increasingly irregular menses, and chronic pelvic pain. Her OBGYN history includes menses onset at nine years old. Her periods are from 24 to 28 days with a 9- to 11-day flow using 5 to 6 pads the first day. A basic introductory history and physical examination were completed. She had some basic lab work drawn and was given an infertility diary to fill out before her next visit.

Case Study

Two weeks later she was seen in the emergency room with high fever, nausea, vomiting, and severe right lower quadrant abdominal pain. She is stoic in her response to pain. Her CBC showed a leukocytosis with a mild bandemia and urine analysis with moderate blood and trace protein. Pelvic ultrasound showed a moderate size pelvic mass in the appendical/tuboovarian region. After a diagnosis of an acute appendicitis was made, she was taken to the operating room. Exploration of the right lower quadrant revealed a strangulated right ovary suspended from a twisted necrotic fallopian tube and diffuse adhesions from the diffuse generalized endometriosis present throughout the right pelvis and abdomen. The surgeons need to perform a right oophorectomy, appendectomy, and adhesion analysis. During the surgery the surgeons also performed some laser coagulation on the numerous endometriosis lesions that were present on the uterus, colon, deep peritoneum, cul-de-sac, omentum, and ipsilateral ovary. Since discharge she has done well and is now here for a six-week postoperative check.

Questions

1. What is endometriosis, and how does it affect the health of the women who develop the disorder?

2. What are the classic signs and symptoms?

3. What is the natural course of endometriosis?

4. What are the different risk factors for the development of endometriosis?

5. What are the different treatment options available for endometriosis?

6. What are chocolate cysts, and how are they treated?

7. Does endometriosis cause cancer?

8. Identify several resources that the nurse can refer Jing to for support.

9. Describe how endometriosis is staged.

10. Are there any natural treatments that have been successful in reducing pain from endometriosis?

Sylvia

AGE

48

SETTING

- Well Women private clinic

CULTURAL CONSIDERATIONS

- Black American professional culture

ETHNICITY

- Black American

PRE-EXISTING CONDITION

- Perimenopause; hypertension

CO-EXISTING CONDITION/CURRENT PROBLEM

- Hypothyroidism; pituitary tumor; obesity; tobacco use; occasional alcohol use

COMMUNICATIONS

DISABILITY

SOCIOECONOMIC STATUS

- Professional

SPIRITUAL/RELIGIOUS

PSYCHOSOCIAL

- Cares for aging mother; work/life balance issues

LEGAL

ETHICAL

PRIORITIZATION

DELEGATION

PHARMACOLOGIC

- Atenolol; fluoxetine (Prozac); calcium; vitamin D

ALTERNATIVE THERAPY

- St. John's wort

SIGNIFICANT HISTORY

- Primipara

WELL WOMAN

Level of difficulty: Moderate

Overview: This case requires that the student be able to assess clinical findings to identify a client with hypothyroidism and potential pituitary tumor. The student is also asked to review prescription medications and possible interactions with the over-the-counter self-medications a client is taking. Finally the student is asked to formulate a care plan complete with teaching.

Client Profile

Sylvia is a 48-year-old, G1P0101, MBF. Her only son is 28 years old and lives in another state. He is married with his own family, and although she is close to her son, they only see each other once a year at Christmas. They do call each other weekly. She has two grandchildren who visit her in the summers for a week. She is divorced and lives with her mother. Her mother suffered a severe stroke ten years ago and she needs assistance with her daily care. During the hours Sylvia works, she has a nursing assistant stay with her mother. After work she assumes full responsibility for caring for her mother. Sylvia is a registered nurse. Currently she is the vice president in charge of nursing at a large teaching hospital. She has 25 years of nursing experience and up until the past two years has been known as a dynamic hands-on leader. Two years ago she experienced a small stroke, which has slowed her down considerably. Although she fully recovered from the stroke, she has found that she no longer has the energy she used to have. She has also gained considerable weight since her stroke. She is five feet three inches tall and her current weight is 168 pounds (BMI 29.8). Sylvia smokes approximately two packs a day and drinks an occasional beer in the late afternoon to relax.

Case Study

Sylvia presents at the Well Woman clinic today for her annual checkup. Her current complaints include lack of energy, noticeable hair loss, weight gain, irregular (every 2 or 3 months) very heavy periods that up until about eight months ago were fairly regular and fairly light, swelling in her feet and ankles at night, and decreasing ability to concentrate. She has started to get headaches that last for several hours and occur at least twice a week. She is not sexually active. She does breast self-exams and states that she has not felt anything unusual, but is worried about a blackish green discharge from her right nipple. After talking to the nurse for a short time she also admits to bouts of depression, which are lasting longer and longer. At today's visit the nurse notes the following: BP 156/88, P 88, R 20; thyroid gland palpable with bruit; skin dry; hair coarse and nails brittle. At her last visit she was prescribed atenolol 50 mg daily to manage her hypertension and fluoxetine (Prozac) 20 mg daily for mild depression.

In an attempt to avoid osteoporosis she takes calcium 1200 mg (600 mg in the morning and 600 mg in the evening) with vitamin D. Because her depression has been getting worse, she also started to take St John's wort 900 mg divided into three doses daily.

Questions

1. Identify at least three possible reasons for Sylvia's weight gain.

2. Make a list of the lab tests that the nurse should anticipate will be ordered for Sylvia at this visit.

3. Give four possible causes for her fatigue.

4. Sylvia has yearly mammograms, does breast self-exams, gets a yearly complete physical, and has no family history of cancer. Using the data from her profile and the case study, assess her risks for breast cancer.

5. How does Sylvia's lifestyle contribute to her chances of having another stroke?

6. How common is thyroid disease in women?

7. Assess her risks for cardiovascular disease.

8. Assess her menstrual changes.

9. Analyze the following lab results:

Cholesterol:
LDL 146 mg/dL
VLDL 41 mg/dL
HDL 33 mg/dL
Triglycerides 207 mg/dL
Total cholesterol 220 mg/dL
TSH 10.2 μIU/mL

10. Sylvia is a Black American woman. How might her race impact on her health risk factors?

11. Many women will self-medicate with over-the-counter medications, herbals, etc. Review her prescription medications and her self-medication and comment on any interactions she needs to be made aware of.

Josephine

AGE

68

SETTING

■ Well Woman clinic

CULTURAL CONSIDERATIONS

■ Advanced age

ETHNICITY

■ White American

PRE-EXISTING CONDITION

■ Malnutrition; asthma

CO-EXISTING CONDITION/CURRENT PROBLEM

■ Osteoporosis

COMMUNICATIONS

■ Not communicating needs with children

DISABILITY

SOCIOECONOMIC STATUS

■ Poverty

SPIRITUAL/RELIGIOUS

■ Catholic

PSYCHOSOCIAL

■ Isolation

LEGAL

ETHICAL

PRIORITIZATION

DELEGATION

PHARMACOLOGIC

■ HRT

ALTERNATIVE THERAPY

SIGNIFICANT HISTORY

■ Multipara; surgical menopause—HRT × 5 years; *Family history:* Heart disease, breast cancer, Alzheimer's disease, and osteoporosis; tobacco use for 20 years

WELL WOMAN

Level of difficulty: Difficult

Overview: Requires knowledge base concerning hormone replacement therapy and menopausal risk for osteoporosis. This case looks at common economic problems facing older woman.

DIFFICULT

121

Client Profile

Josephine is a 68-year-old, G3P3003, widowed, white female. She breastfed all of her children for one year. Her last physical exam was three years ago. At that time she was five feet, five inches tall and weighed 110 lbs.

Family History: Mother died of a heart attack at age 82; father is living but has Alzheimer's and is living in a complete care facility. She has two sisters; one is 72 and is very healthy except for some minor problems with osteoporosis, and the other one is 76 and is fighting the final stages of breast cancer. She takes short walks, but lately she has been afraid to walk alone since there have been some muggings of older people in her neighborhood. Her children have encouraged her to come live with them to get away from her changing neighborhood, but she has many good memories of her husband there and does not want to leave her home. Besides, she does not want to become a burden to her children. She has a dog, who is now 12 years old, and a cat, 13 years old, as her only companions. She is very attached to her pets.

Medical History: Asthma as a child and into the teens. She smoked one pack of cigarettes a day for 20 years, but quit 14 years ago, when she could not afford it anymore.

Surgical History: Hysterectomy and oophorectomy at age 48 for menometrorrhagia. She took HRT for five years for hot flashes and mood swings and then decided to discontinue them herself.

Psychosocial History: She is living on a diminishing income. Her husband died four years ago after a long fight with lung cancer. With his death, her income dropped to half. She has Medicare but cannot afford the supplemental coverage. Her children do not know how financially needy she is, and she will not tell them. She says, "They all have children in college and they need their money." Some days she is only able to eat one meal and often that meal is a bowl of cereal. She does make sure that her pets eat each day.

Case Study

Today Josephine is being seen in the Well Woman clinic for progressively worsening backache. On exam her height is five feet three inches and her weight is 106 pounds.

Questions

1. Identify at least three health risks for Josephine and give at least two pieces of supporting data for each of your choices.

2. How does her history of breastfeeding for three years affect her risk for osteoporosis?

3. How does breastfeeding affect her risk for breast cancer today?

4. Define menometrorrhagia.

5. Does Josephine need a PAP smear today?

6. What other screening tests are appropriate for her at this visit?

7. How does surgical menopause differ from natural menopause?

8. What effect does her five years on HRT have on her health risk for heart disease?

9. What effect does her five years on HRT have on her health risk for osteoporosis?

10. What resources can you suggest to help with her financial and living situation?

11. Develop a teaching plan to help Josephine minimize her health risk.

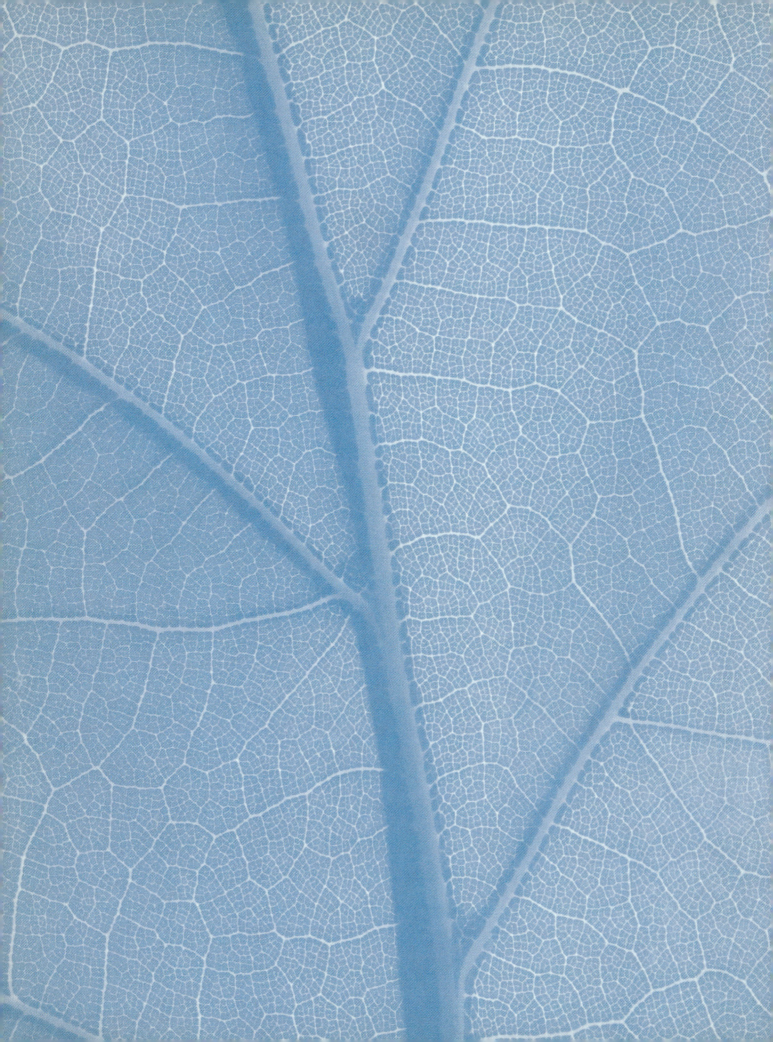

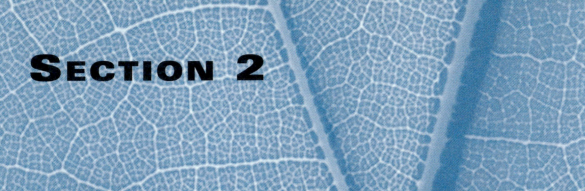

SECTION 2

CLINICAL DECISION MAKING

Case Studies in Pediatrics

Bonita Broyles
RN, BSN, MA, PhD

Instructor
ADN PROGRAM, PIEDMONT COMMUNITY COLLEGE,
NORTH CAROLINA

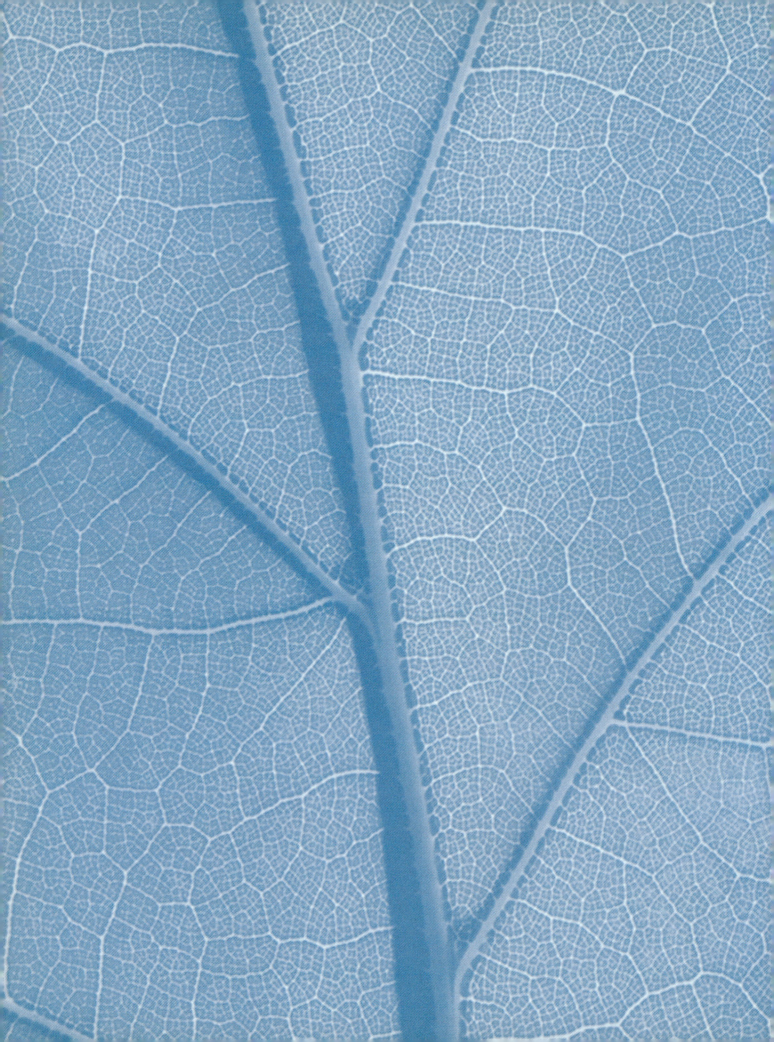

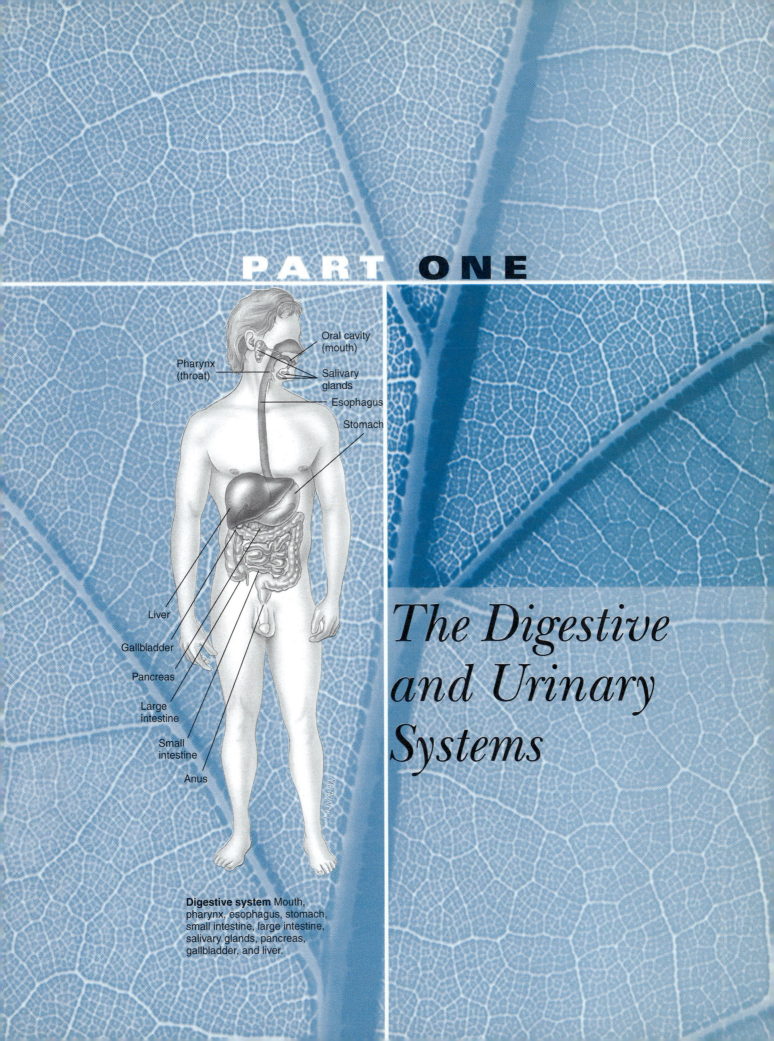

PART ONE

Oral cavity
(mouth)

Pharynx
(throat)

Salivary
glands

Esophagus

Stomach

Liver

Gallbladder

Pancreas

Large
intestine

Small
intestine

Anus

Digestive system Mouth,
pharynx, esophagus, stomach,
small intestine, large intestine,
salivary glands, pancreas,
gallbladder, and liver.

*The Digestive
and Urinary
Systems*

CASE STUDY 1

Shelly

GENDER

F

AGE

4

SETTING

- Home/clinic

ETHNICITY

- White American

CULTURAL CONSIDERATIONS

PREEXISTING CONDITIONS

COEXISTING CONDITIONS

SIGNIFICANT HISTORY

COMMUNICATION

DISABILITY

SOCIOECONOMIC

SPIRITUAL

PHARMACOLOGIC

- Acetominaphen (Tylenol)
- Trimephoprim-Sulfamethoxazole (Bactrim)

PSYCHOSOCIAL

- Fear

LEGAL

ETHICAL

ALTERNATIVE THERAPY

PRIORITIZATION

- Yes

DELEGATION

- Client teaching

THE URINARY SYSTEM

Level of difficulty: Easy

Overview: This case requires knowledge of urinary tract infections, growth and development, as well as understanding of the client's background, personal situation, and parent–child relationship.

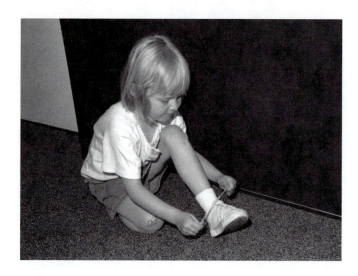

Client Profile

Shelly is a 4-year-old preschooler who lives with her parents and younger brother. She and her brother attend a local daycare center during the week while their parents are at work. In the evenings she and her brother take a bath and then their parents read to them before bedtime at 8:00 P.M. Shelly's daycare class includes many children her age and she enjoys playing outside with them. Although snack times are planned, Shelly would rather play and does not always finish her beverages.

Case Study

Shelly's mother calls the pediatric clinic in town and tells the nurse that Shelly has been "running a fever of 101° F for the past 2 days" and although her temperature decreases to 37.2° C (99° F) with acetaminophen, it returns to 38.4° C, (101° F) within 4 hours of each dose. Further, her mother says that Shelly complains that "it hurts when I pee-pee." Shelly's mother also has noticed that her daughter seems to be in the bathroom "every hour." She makes an appointment to see the pediatrician this afternoon.

Questions

1. Discuss the significance of Shelly's clinical manifestations.

2. What other assessment data would be helpful for the nurse to have to prepare Shelly's care plan?

3. Discuss Shelly's anatomic risk factor(s) for developing a urinary tract infection (UTI).

4. Discuss the relationship between Shelly's hygiene habits and her risk for developing a UTI.

5. Discuss how Shelly's level of growth and development places her at risk for developing a UTI.

6. Shelly's urine culture returns positive for *Escherichia coli*. What is the significance of this finding?

7. What are the priorities for Shelly's care?

8. Shelly is prescribed trimethoprim-sulfamethoxazole 60 mg every 12 hours for 10 days. What is this drug and is her prescribed dose safe? Shelly weighs 33 lb.

9. What are the teaching priorities for Shelly and her mother prior to her discharge from the clinic?

10. Shelly is scheduled for a return visit to the clinic in 2 weeks. What is the purpose of this appointment?

Justin

GENDER	
M	
AGE	
Neonate	
SETTING	
■ Hospital	
ETHNICITY	
■ White American	
CULTURAL CONSIDERATIONS	
PREEXISTING CONDITIONS	
COEXISTING CONDITIONS	
SIGNIFICANT HISTORY	
COMMUNICATION	
DISABILITY	

SOCIOECONOMIC	
SPIRITUAL	
PHARMACOLOGIC	
PSYCHOSOCIAL	
■ No prenatal care	
■ Teenage mother	
LEGAL	
ETHICAL	
ALTERNATIVE THERAPY	
PRIORITIZATION	
■ Yes	
DELEGATION	

MODERATE

THE DIGESTIVE SYSTEM

Level of difficulty: Moderate

Overview: This case requires knowledge of the impact of TEF, growth and development on mother and son, as well as an understanding of the client's background, personal situation, and mother–child attachment relationship.

Client Profile

Justin is a neonate whose mother, Danielle, is a 16-year-old young woman who lives at home with her mother and 14-year-old sister. Danielle is in her 36th week of pregnancy and has not received any prenatal care because "we can't afford it." She stopped going to school last month because she was self-conscious of her appearance. The father of her unborn child does not live in the area, and from the time she told him of the pregnancy he has shown no interest in her or the unborn child.

Case Study

Danielle is admitted to the hospital in active labor, and 10 hours later Justin is born. His Apgar score is 4 at 1 minute and 6 at 5 minutes. He is cyanotic and coughing, and chokes on his oral secretions. He is admitted to the nursery and examined by the pediatrician on call. He is diagnosed with tracheoesophageal fistula (TEF) and transferred to the pediatric intensive care unit for monitoring. He is scheduled for surgery to repair his TEF.

Questions

1. What is the meaning of Justin's Apgar score?

2. Discuss esophageal atresia and TEF.

3. How common is TEF and what causes it?

4. How is TEF diagnosed?

5. Discuss the problems associated with Justin's mother not receiving prenatal care.

6. Identify the priority nursing concerns for Justin.

7. Discuss the appropriate priority nursing interventions for Justin.

8. Because of Justin's condition, Danielle has had difficulty bonding with him. Discuss the concept of bonding (attachment) and your impressions of its importance.

9. Justin's TEF is surgically repaired when he is 1 day old and a D-tube is placed. Why would Justin require enteral feedings during his surgical recovery?

10. Danielle was discharged when Justin was 2 days old. She visited him once a day with her mother. Justin is 5 days postop and with an anticipated discharge in 2 days. How can the nurse assist with maternal–infant bonding and prepare Danielle for Justin's care at home?

Beth

GENDER	**SOCIOECONOMIC**
F	■ Middle class
AGE	**SPIRITUAL**
4 months	
SETTING	**PHARMACOLOGIC**
■ Clinic	
ETHNICITY	**PSYCHOSOCIAL**
■ White American	■ Parental anxiety
CULTURAL CONSIDERATIONS	■ Caregiver stress
	■ Breastfeeding support
PREEXISTING CONDITIONS	**LEGAL**
■ Preterm birth	
COEXISTING CONDITIONS	**ETHICAL**
SIGNIFICANT HISTORY	**ALTERNATIVE THERAPY**
COMMUNICATION	**PRIORITIZATION**
	■ Yes
DISABILITY	**DELEGATION**
	■ Yes

MODERATE

THE DIGESTIVE SYSTEM

Level of difficulty: Moderate

Overview: This case requires knowledge of infant feeding, association between preterm birth and gastroesophageal reflux as well as an understanding of the client's background, personal situation, and mother–child attachment relationship.

Client Profile

Beth is a 4-month-old infant who was delivered by Cesarean section at 35 weeks' gestation, weighing 2.3 kg (5 lb) and measuring 42.5 cm (17 in.) in length. She is the first child for Robert and Janice Carter. Since birth Beth has been a "fussy" baby who frequently "throws up after almost every feeding and cries all the time." Janice stays home and cares for Beth while Robert works; however, when he comes home from work each day, he helps with Beth's care. Beth is clean and obviously well cared for by her parents, who appear to have bonded well with her and love her very much. During her recent 4-month check-up Beth was diagnosed with gastro-esophageal reflux (GER) following a battery of diagnostic tests in response to Beth's history of frequent regurgitation following feedings. Janice's parents live in the same town as Janice and Robert and his parents live a 30-minute driving distance away.

Case Study

Janice and Robert bring Beth in for a 2-week weight check at the pediatrician's office. During the nurse's family assessment, Janice and Robert appear exhausted and anxious. Janice comments, "I feel like it's my fault that Beth is not gaining weight as she should. I get so frustrated because she is still throwing up after at least two breastfeedings a day. I try but I don't think I'm a very good mother. Maybe I should give up breastfeeding and give her a bottle." Robert further states that his family has a history of gastric ulcer disease and asked if he "gave this stomach problem to her." The couple comment that they are not sure they are doing the right things for Beth and question how they are going to manage caring for her. At this visit Beth weighs 3.4 kg (7.5 lb), her posterior fontanel is closed, and her anterior fontanel remains opened and level with suture lines.

Questions

1. Discuss your impressions about the above situation.

2. What is the incidence and etiology of GER in children?

3. How does GER differ from pyloric stenosis?

4. Identify the priority nursing concerns for Beth and her parents.

5. Discuss the nurse's findings concerning Beth's fontanels.

6. Discuss the relationship between Beth being preterm, her birth weight, and her current weight.

7. How would you respond to Janice's concern about breastfeeding and Beth's GER?

8. During the nurse's assessment of Beth's growth and development, she finds that Beth can put her hand to her mouth, lift her head up from a prone position, turn and look for sounds, focus on the face of the person speaking to her, and that the head lag is present when she is pulled to sitting position. Beth's rooting reflex is not present, nor is the moro reflex and tonic neck. Her sucking reflex is still present as well as her step, Babinski, ciliary, and grasp reflexes. How would you interpret these findings?

9. How would you respond to Janice and Robert's concerns about how Beth developed GER and their feelings of blame?

10. Discuss the teaching plan for Beth and her parents.

11. What suggestions could you offer Janice and Robert to provide them with support as they care for Beth at home?

CASE STUDY 4

Jesus

GENDER	**SOCIOECONOMIC**
M	■ Lower socioeconomic
AGE	**SPIRITUAL**
4	
SETTING	**PHARMACOLOGIC**
■ Hospital	■ Acetaminophen (Tylenol)
ETHNICITY	■ Morphine sulfate (Duromorph)
■ Mexican American	■ Gentamicin (Garamycin)
	■ Ampicillin sodium /Sulbactam sodium (Unasyn)
CULTURAL CONSIDERATIONS	**PSYCHOSOCIAL**
■ Hispanic	■ Client anxiety
PREEXISTING CONDITIONS	■ Parental anxiety
	LEGAL
COEXISTING CONDITIONS	■ Informed consent
	ETHICAL
SIGNIFICANT HISTORY	
	ALTERNATIVE THERAPY
COMMUNICATION	
■ Spanish-speaking	**PRIORITIZATION**
DISABILITY	■ Emergency room care
	DELEGATION
	■ Yes

THE DIGESTIVE SYSTEM

Level of difficulty: Moderate

Overview: This case requires knowledge of appendicitis, growth and development, stressors of hospitalization on children and parents, and appendicitis treatment.

135

Client Profile

Jesus is a 5-year-old boy who recently moved to the United States with his mother, 7-year-old sister Carleen, and 14-year-old brother Juan to join his father, who is employed as a worker in a packaging company. Mr. Rodriquez joined the company 1 year ago and has been saving money to send for his family. During his employment, Mr. Rodriquez has learned to speak and understand English by taking an "English as a Second Language" course at the local community college. Except for 14-year-old Juan, who has been studying English so he can enter school in the fall, Mr. Rodriquez's wife and children do not speak or understand English. Mrs. Rodriquez plans to attend the same community college as her husband so she can learn to speak English. Jesus' parents are excited to have the family together in their new home, and Jesus and his sister have met a few of the neighborhood children and enjoy playing with them even though the other children are English speaking.

Case Study

Jesus wakes up at 2:00 A.M. crying, telling his mother his "stomach hurts." He has an elevated temperature of 37.9° C (100.2° F) and begins to vomit. His parents administer 120 mg of acetaminophen orally; however, Jesus has emesis 5 minutes later. They continue to monitor him for an hour and then Mr. Rodriquez decides he and his wife should take Jesus to the local hospital emergency room. Mr. Rodriquez wakes Juan and explains that Jesus has to go to the hospital and that Juan must take care of Carleen until one of his parents returns home. Jesus is admitted through the emergency department. On admission Jesus' vital signs are: axillary temperature, 38° C (100.4° F); pulse, 125 beats/minute; respirations, 35 breaths/minute; blood pressure, 119/79; weight, 18.3 kg (40.3 lb); height, 111 cm (44.4 in.). Jesus guards the lower right quadrant of his abdomen and is crying. An intravenous access is established and morphine sulfate 2.0 mg is administered IV for pain control. An abdominal ultrasound is prescribed to confirm his suspected diagnosis. Jesus' leukocyte count is 17,500 cells/mm³.

Questions

1. Discuss your impressions about the above situation including pathophysiology and potential complications.

2. Compare Jesus' vital signs, height, and weight to the normal readings for a child his age and discuss the possible reasons for any abnormal values.

3. Calculate the safe dosage ranges for the acetaminophen his parents administer and the morphine sulfate administered in the emergency department to determine whether he received safe doses of these two medications.

4. The abdominal ultrasound confirms that Jesus has appendicitis. Discuss the following prescription of treatment by the care provider:

    a. Bedrest

    b. NPO

    c. Intravenous fluids of D_5 and .45% normal saline with 10 mEq of potassium chloride at 70 mL/hour.

    d. Gentamicin 45 mg IV on call to operating room

    e. Morphine sulfate 2 mg IV q1–2h PRN pain

    f. K-pad to abdomen

    g. Prepare for OR for laparoscopic appendectomy

5. The preoperative instructions are given to Mr. Rodriquez, who in turn translates them for his wife and Jesus. Mr. and Mrs. Rodriquez give informed consent and Jesus assents to the surgery after his father explains the procedure to him. How does informed consent of the parents differ from Jesus' assent?

6. Why is it important to include Jesus in the surgical consent?

7. Just prior to a his transfer to a holding area before surgery, Jesus experiences a sudden relief of pain that is followed by an increase in pain. What is your impression of this and what is your first action?

8. Jesus undergoes an exploratory laparotomy and appendectomy. Discuss the nursing priorities as he recovers from anesthesia.

9. Mr. and Mrs. Rodriquez are present in the PACU when Jesus awakens from anesthesia. Discuss the pros and cons of allowing parents in the PACU when children awake from anesthesia.

10. After Jesus is transferred to his room on your nursing unit at 5 A.M., Mr. Rodriquez states that he must leave to check on their other children and then must go to work. He says he will return after he finishes work and prepares dinner for Juan and Carlene. How will you communicate with Jesus and his mother in Mr. Rodriquez's absence?

11. Discuss how you think you would feel if you were in Mrs. Rodriquez's position with your child in the hospital following surgery and you were unable to speak the language.

12. The transfer orders on Jesus include the following:

   a. Routine postoperative vital signs

   b. Foley catheter to straight drain

   c. D_5 and .45% normal saline with 20 mEq of potassium chloride at 75 mL/hour. Medlock when urine output adequate and taking fluids well.

   d. Gentamicin sulfate 45 mg IV q8h

   e. Ampicillin sodium/sulbactam sodium 900 mg IV q6h

   f. Morphine sulfate 0.5 mg continuous IV and 0.5 mg patient-controlled analgesia

   g. Acetaminophen 240 mg q4h per N/G tube for temperature > 37.5° C (99.5° F)

   h. NPO except medications

   i. Nasogastric tube (Salem sump) to continuous wall suction

   j. Incentive spirometry 10 times each hour while awake

   k. Notify house officer for temperature >38° C (100.4° F).

Discuss the nursing interventions involved in Jesus's care.

Jamal

GENDER

M

AGE

18 months old

SETTING

- Hospital

ETHNICITY

- Black American

CULTURAL CONSIDERATIONS

PREEXISTING CONDITIONS

- Short bowel syndrome

COEXISTING CONDITIONS

SIGNIFICANT HISTORY

- Single grandmother

COMMUNICATION

DISABILITY

SOCIOECONOMIC

- Middle class
- Single parent

SPIRITUAL

PHARMACOLOGIC

PSYCHOSOCIAL

- Parental anxiety
- Grandmother is caregiver

LEGAL

ETHICAL

ALTERNATIVE THERAPY

PRIORITIZATION

- Yes

DELEGATION

THE DIGESTIVE SYSTEM

Level of difficulty: Moderate

Overview: This case requires knowledge of short bowel syndrome and total parenteral nutrition, as well as an understanding of the client's background, personal situation, and family dynamics.

Client Profile

Jamal is an 18-month-old toddler who was born with short bowel syndrome (SBS), weighed 3.2 kg (7 lb), and was 50 cm (19.7 in.) in length at birth. He has lived with his grandmother since his discharge from the hospital 10 months after birth. He has a central venous access device (CVAD) through which he receives home total parenteral nutrition (TPN). His lengthy hospitalization resulted from the severity of his short bowel syndrome; Jamal was born with only 40 cm (15.8 in.) of intestine secondary to jejunal–ileal atresia. He experienced recurrent respiratory infections. Initially his parents visited him every day; however, his father was transferred in his job to a city 3 hours driving distance away when Jamal was 3 months old. Since that time, the parents' visits became infrequent and eventually they gave custody of Jamal to his grandmother because "they just couldn't handle his care." His grandmother has been a very attentive guardian and is very involved in his care. She works for a company that allows her to work from home so she can care for Jamal.

Case Study

Jamal's grandmother brings him to the emergency department of the children's hospital located in the city where they live because of recurrent episodes of fever, irritability, and "temper tantrums." Today the site of his central venous access device (CVAD) was reddened with "some discharge" under the dressing. Jamal is admitted to the pediatric medical nursing unit. His grandmother is very concerned about Jamal's condition and the fact that he required hospitalization. She verbalizes that she feels she is to blame for his current condition. The nurse's assessment reveals the following:

Temperature: 38.6° C (101.5° F)

Pulse: 120 beats/minute

Respirations: 30 breaths/minute

Height: 75 cm (30 in.)

Weight: 10 kg (22 lb)

Questions

1. Discuss your impressions about the above situation.

2. What additional data would be helpful for the nurse to have to develop Jamal's plan of care?

3. Discuss the pathophysiology of short bowel syndrome.

4. What is Jamal's prognosis for being weaned from TPN and developing a functional intestine?

5. Discuss TPN, including indications for use.

6. Why is Jamal at risk for infection?

7. Jamal's TPN solution has completed; however, the next bag of TPN has not arrived from the pharmacy. What actions should you take at this time?

8. Identify the priorities of care for Jamal.

9. Discuss the nursing interventions that are critical in preventing infection when caring for Jamal.

10. How do you as the nurse explain Jamal's "temper tantrums" to his grandmother?

11. How will you evaluate Jamal's grandmother's ability to care for Jamal at home?

Kurt

GENDER	**SOCIOECONOMIC**
M	
AGE	**SPIRITUAL**
2 days old	
SETTING	**PHARMACOLOGIC**
■ Hospital	■ Acetaminophen (Tylenol)
ETHNICITY	**PSYCHOSOCIAL**
■ White American	■ Parental anxiety
CULTURAL CONSIDERATIONS	**LEGAL**
PREEXISTING CONDITIONS	**ETHICAL**
COEXISTING CONDITIONS	**ALTERNATIVE THERAPY**
SIGNIFICANT HISTORY	**PRIORITIZATION**
	■ Yes
COMMUNICATION	**DELEGATION**
	■ Yes
DISABILITY	

THE DIGESTIVE SYSTEM

Level of difficulty: Moderate

Overview: This case requires knowledge of imperforate anus; anal atresia; colostomy care; growth and development; and an understanding of the client's background, personal situation, and parent–child relationship.

Client Profile   **Kurt** is a neonate who weighed 3.5 kg (7 lb, 11 oz) at birth and was 20 in. (50 cm) long. He is the first child for Karen and Kevin. Karen had an uneventful pregnancy and delivery and breastfed Kurt immediately after birth. Kurt also is the first grandson for both sets of grandparents, who saw him immediately after he was born in the birthing room of the hospital. Kevin has taken paternity leave from his job to stay home with Kurt and Karen for 6 weeks.

Case Study   Within 24 hours of his birth, Kurt is examined by the pediatrician, who determines Kurt has imperforate anus. Following diagnostic testing, the diagnosis is confirmed and Karen and Kevin are informed by the pediatrician that Kurt has a high anal defect that will require surgery and the formation of a colostomy. They are devastated and express concern for their son "going through surgery when he is so young." Kurt's surgery is scheduled for the following day.

Questions

1. How should the nurse respond to Karen and Kevin's concerns?

2. Discuss imperforate anus, its incidence, and cause.

3. Kurt's parents ask the nurse why Kurt has to have a colostomy. How should the nurse respond?

4. Karen expresses concern about the impact the surgery will have on her ability to breastfeed Kurt. What is the nurse's most appropriate response to Karen's concern?

5. Kurt undergoes an anoplasty and a transverse colostomy. What are the priorities for his care following surgery and his return to the pediatric nursing unit?

6. What precautions should be taken when caring for Kurt following surgery?

7. Kurt's surgeon prescribes acetaminophen for Kurt's postoperative pain. Discuss your impressions of this and the appropriate actions the nurse should take.

8. Kurt's recovery allows him to be discharged to his parents. Discuss the parental teaching necessary for Karen and Kevin prior to Kurt's discharge.

9. Kurt is now 2 months old and returns to have a colostomy takedown. He has been breastfeeding well and the skin around his colostomy is clean and dry without any evidence of excoriation. What are your impressions of Kurt's present condition?

10. What assessment should the nurse include in her care of Kurt following surgery?

Nathan

GENDER	**SOCIOECONOMIC**
M	
AGE	**SPIRITUAL**
6	
SETTING	**PHARMACOLOGIC**
Hospital	■ Nitazoxanide (Alinia)
ETHNICITY	**PSYCHOSOCIAL**
■ Black American	■ Fear/anxiety
CULTURAL CONSIDERATIONS	**LEGAL**
PREEXISTING CONDITIONS	**ETHICAL**
COEXISTING CONDITIONS	**ALTERNATIVE THERAPY**
■ Diarrhea	
SIGNIFICANT HISTORY	**PRIORITIZATION**
	■ Yes
COMMUNICATION	**DELEGATION**
	■ Client teaching
DISABILITY	

THE DIGESTIVE SYSTEM

Level of difficulty: Moderate

Overview: This case requires knowledge of diarrhea, acid–base imbalances, fluid and electrolyte balance, client teaching, as well as an understanding of the client's background, personal situation, and mother–child attachment relationship, and of growth and development of the school-age child.

Client Profile

Nathan is a 6-year-old first grader who lives with his mother and older brother, 8-year-old Micah. Nathan has been a healthy child with only occasional upper respiratory infections. His mother diligently kept up with his immunizations and all of his pediatric check-ups. He started first grade 2 weeks ago and is always eager to go to school. His level of growth and development is appropriate for his age and he quickly developed friendships with his classmates.

Case Study

Yesterday afternoon when he came home from school, Nathan began having episodes of abdominal pain and diarrhea. His stools have been intermittent, foul smelling, watery, and, according to Nathan's mother, "float in the toilet." He refused to eat or drink anything since that time so Nathan's mother calls the pediatrician. At the pediatrician's office Nathan is listless, his skin is warm and dry, and he complains that his "tummy hurts." His urine specific gravity is 1.040, his heart rate is 120 beats/minute, his respirations are 30 breaths/minute, and his blood pressure is 78/46. His stool is negative for blood and his complete blood count results are as follows:

Hematocrit: 50%

Hemoglobin: 16.5 g/dL

Platelets: 455,000 cells/mm^3

Red blood cell count: 5.2 million cells/mm^3

White blood cell count: 11,300 cells/mm^3

Because he continues to refuse to eat or drink, the pediatrician recommends that he be hospitalized for further diagnostic testing.

Questions

1. Discuss your impressions about the above situation.

2. Because of Nathan's symptoms, the pediatrician prescribes arterial blood gases (ABGs) be drawn. What is the purpose of this prescription and what nursing implications are appropriate prior to drawing Nathan's ABGs?

3. Nathan's ABG results are: pH, 7.30; Pco$_2$, 30 mm Hg; Po$_2$, 90 mm Hg; oxygen saturation, 94%; and bicarbonate (HCO$_3$), 22 mEq/L. Compare his values to the normal values for a child Nathan's age.

4. Discuss Nathan's blood gas values considering his present condition and clinical manifestations.

5. What is the significance of Nathan's hematological test results and his urine specific gravity?

6. What additional data would be helpful in confirming Nathan's diagnosis?

7. Nathan is diagnosed with giardiasis and is prescribed nitazoxanide. What is this agent and would you question it being prescribed for Nathan?

8. What are the nursing priorities for Nathan's case?

9. Nathan begins to respond to therapy and is beginning to eat and drink. What play activities would be appropriate for Nathan while he is hospitalized?

10. What are the teaching priorities you should discuss with Nathan's mother prior to his discharge?

GENDER

F

AGE

Neonate

SETTING

■ Hospital

ETHNICITY

■ Spanish American

CULTURAL CONSIDERATIONS

PREEXISTING CONDITIONS

COEXISTING CONDITIONS

SIGNIFICANT HISTORY

COMMUNICATION

DISABILITY

SOCIOECONOMIC

SPIRITUAL

PHARMACOLOGIC

PSYCHOSOCIAL

■ Potential impaired parent—infant attachment

LEGAL

ETHICAL

ALTERNATIVE THERAPY

PRIORITIZATION

■ Yes

DELEGATION

■ Yes

MODERATE

THE DIGESTIVE SYSTEM

Level of difficulty: Moderate

Overview: This case requires knowledge of cleft lip/cleft palate (CL/CP) surgical repair, growth and development, and parent–child attachment relationship.

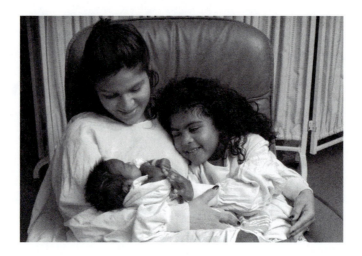

Client Profile

Marissa is a newborn weighing 14.2 kg (6 lb, 7 oz) who was born with a cleft lip and palate. She is the third child of Juan and Maria.

Case Study

When Marissa is first brought from the nursery to Maria's room, Maria and Juan are visually alarmed at Marissa's appearance. The nurse notes that Maria holds her daughter in her lap, looking at her while Juan moves from the bedside to a chair next to the bed. Maria begins to cry, "My poor baby. What will happen to her? Everyone will make fun of her. What have we done to her?"

Questions

1. Discuss your impressions of this situation.

2. What is the incidence and etiology of cleft lip and cleft palate?

3. Is the response seen in Marissa's parents unusual?

4. How can the nurse therapeutically respond to Maria and Juan?

5. Discuss the standard of care for the surgical repair of Marissa's cleft lip and cleft palate.

6. What are the current priorities of care for Marissa?

7. Discuss the impact of Marissa's defect on her growth and development.

8. Discuss the teaching priorities for Marissa's parents prior to her discharge at 5 days of age.

9. Marissa returns to the hospital at 8 weeks of age for the surgical repair of her cleft lip. What are the priorities of care for Marissa following her surgery?

10. Discuss the nursing interventions to meet Marissa's care needs.

11. Even following Marissa's cleft palate repair, her parents note that she still does not "talk much" and when she does, it is "difficult to understand her. Our other children were very talkative by this age. What should we do?" What actions should the nurse take?

Sandra

GENDER	**SOCIOECONOMIC**
F	
AGE	**SPIRITUAL**
14	
SETTING	**PHARMACOLOGIC**
■ Home/clinic/hospital	■ Prednisone (Deltasone)
ETHNICITY	■ Cyclosporine (Restasis)
	■ Azathioprine (Azasan)
■ White American	**PSYCHOSOCIAL**
CULTURAL CONSIDERATIONS	■ Fear/anxiety
	LEGAL
PREEXISTING CONDITIONS	
■ Motor vehicle accident	**ETHICAL**
■ Acute renal failure	
COEXISTING CONDITIONS	**ALTERNATIVE THERAPY**
SIGNIFICANT HISTORY	**PRIORITIZATION**
	■ Yes
COMMUNICATION	**DELEGATION**
DISABILITY	

THE URINARY SYSTEM

Level of difficulty: Moderate

Overview: This case requires knowledge of acute renal failure and associated complications; growth and development; as well as an understanding of the client's background, personal situation, and family–child relationship.

Client Profile

Sandra is a 14-year-old adolescent who lives at home with her mother, step-father, and two younger siblings. When Sandra was 9 years old, she was involved in a motor vehicle accident and severely injured. As a result, she developed acute renal failure that eventually progressed to chronic renal failure. She has been receiving peritoneal dialysis for the past 4 years. She is registered with the organ procurement agency in the city 30 miles from her home because her parents have been ruled out as potential donors.

Case Study

Sandra is doing satisfactorily at home, receiving her peritoneal dialysis at night. This allows her to attend school and interact with her friends. She is anxious to receive a kidney transplant so she will not have to continue her dialysis. Sandra's parents receive a phone call from the hospital at 2 o'clock A.M. telling them that the hospital has procured a kidney for Sandra as a result of a motor vehicle crash that killed a 10-year-old boy. Her mother calls Sandra's grandmother to babysit for the younger siblings, and then Sandra's parents take her to the hospital, where they are met by the transplant team.

Questions

1. What is chronic renal failure and End-Stage Renal Disease (ESRD)?

2. Discuss the possible connection between Sandra's motor vehicle accident and her development of ESRD.

3. Discuss the incidence and etiology of chronic renal failure in children.

4. Discuss the complications associated with Sandra's diagnosis.

5. What are the priorities of care for Sandra's ESRD?

6. Why is Sandra receiving peritoneal dialysis?

7. Compare the advantages and disadvantages of peritoneal dialysis and hemodialysis in children.

8. Discuss the impact Sandra's diagnosis may have on her growth and development.

9. What other assessment data would be helpful for the nurse to have to prepare Sandra's care plan?

10. Discuss the impact of the phone call Sandra's parents received informing them of a kidney donor for Sandra.

11. What is the incidence of renal transplants in a child of Sandra's age?

12. Two days following her surgery, Sandra is admitted to the pediatric transplant unit where she received her kidney transplant. What are the priority nursing interventions for Sandra?

13. Sandra weighs 110 lb and is prescribed prednisone 30 mg by mouth q.i.d., cyclosporine 100 mg by mouth q.i.d., and azathioprine 50 mg by mouth q.i.d. Discuss these medications and if they are safe for Sandra in the doses prescribed.

14. One month following Sandra's discharge from the hospital, she develops a fever, has decreased urine output, and has gained 3.2 kg (7 lb). Her mother calls Sandra's transplant physician and is advised to bring Sandra to the hospital clinic. On arrival her vital signs are: temperature, 38° C (100.4° F); pulse, 90 beats/minute; respirations, 30 breaths/minute; and blood pressure, 140/86. Her blood urea nitrogen (BUN) is 24 mg/dL and her creatinine is 4 mg/dL. Discuss your impressions of Sandra's condition.

15. Sandra is admitted to the hospital and prescribed prednisone 40 mg by mouth q.i.d, cyclosporine 125 mg by mouth q.i.d., and azathioprine 62.5 mg by mouth q.i.d. Discuss the relationship between Sandra's condition and the increase in her medications.

16. Sandra's acute rejection is successfully treated and she returns home. Three years later Sandra is doing well and her transplanted kidney is functioning well. Does Sandra need to continue her immunosuppressant therapy? If so, for how long?

Cammie

GENDER	**SOCIOECONOMIC**
F	■ Upper class
AGE	**SPIRITUAL**
14	
SETTING	**PHARMACOLOGIC**
■ Hospital	
ETHNICITY	**PSYCHOSOCIAL**
■ White American	
CULTURAL CONSIDERATIONS	**LEGAL**
PREEXISTING CONDITIONS	**ETHICAL**
	■ Potential nurse bias
COEXISTING CONDITIONS	**ALTERNATIVE THERAPY**
SIGNIFICANT HISTORY	**PRIORITIZATION**
	■ Yes
COMMUNICATION	**DELEGATION**
DISABILITY	

DIFFICULT

THE DIGESTIVE SYSTEM

Level of difficulty: Difficult

Overview: This case requires knowledge of eating disorders, growth, and development; understanding of the client's background, personal situation, and parent–child relationship.

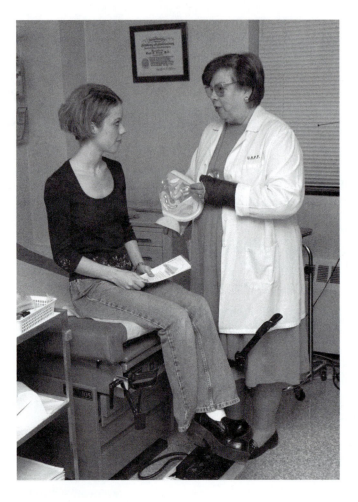

Client Profile

Cammie is a 14-year-old adolescent who lives with her mother. Her mother and father were divorced 3 years ago, and she sees her father every other week. Cammie has lost 15.9 kg (35 lb) since her physical exam last year. Despite the weight loss, Cammie has continued to go to school, making the A honor roll. She jogs 2 miles a day regardless of the weather. Her mother works and frequently is not home at dinner time, leaving Cammie to prepare her own dinner. Cammie packs her own lunch for school and often only drinks orange juice for breakfast before leaving for school. She seldom goes out with her friends; however, she talks to her 15-year-old boyfriend on the phone every evening. She weighs herself every morning at the same time, making sure she is unclothed when she gets on the scale. She experienced menarche at the age of 11, but has not had menses for the past 6 months.

Case Study

Cammie's mother accompanies her to her annual physical. Her pediatrician notes that Cammie is small for her age and looks younger than her years. She brings with her a bottle of water and drinks frequently during the visit. During the examination, she denies dizziness or fainting spells and states she feels "fine." When asked about her diet, Cammie becomes indignant, saying, "I eat when I'm hungry, but I watch what I eat because I'm fat." Her vital signs are within normal limits for her age and she denies using either drugs or alcohol. Because of the pediatrician's concern, he recommends that Cammie be admitted to the adolescent psychiatric unit at the city hospital. Her mother and father accompany her during her admission.

Questions

1. Discuss your impressions of the above situation.

2. Discuss the significance of Cammie's clinical manifestations.

3. What other assessment data would be helpful for the nurse to have to prepare Cammie's care plan?

4. Discuss the difference between anorexia and bulimia.

5. During the interview with Cammie, the nurse notes that Cammie is distant and terse in her answers concerning her perception of herself; however, the teen does confirm that she thinks she is "fat." What is the relationship between body image, need for control, and eating disorders?

6. What are the priorities of care for Cammie on admission?

7. During the interview with Cammie's parents, the nurse notes that both are well dressed and very successful in their respective careers. They state that they have given Cammie "everything." Neither is aware of what Cammie eats or her daily schedule outside of school because they believe that "girls her age need privacy and we try to honor that. Her mother was neither aware nor concerned about Cammie's lack of menses. Both parents exercise regularly and believe that daily exercise and "eating right" is the "key to good health." They both state that they are very proud of Cammie and do not understand the pediatrician's concern. Further, they deny that Cammie has ever had any psychiatric problems. Discuss your impressions of this interview and the possible relationship with Cammie's eating disorder.

8. Discuss your impression of the communication within this family.

9. Discuss your biases about adolescents and eating disorders.

10. Given your biases, if any, how can you intervene to address the nursing priorities for Cammie?

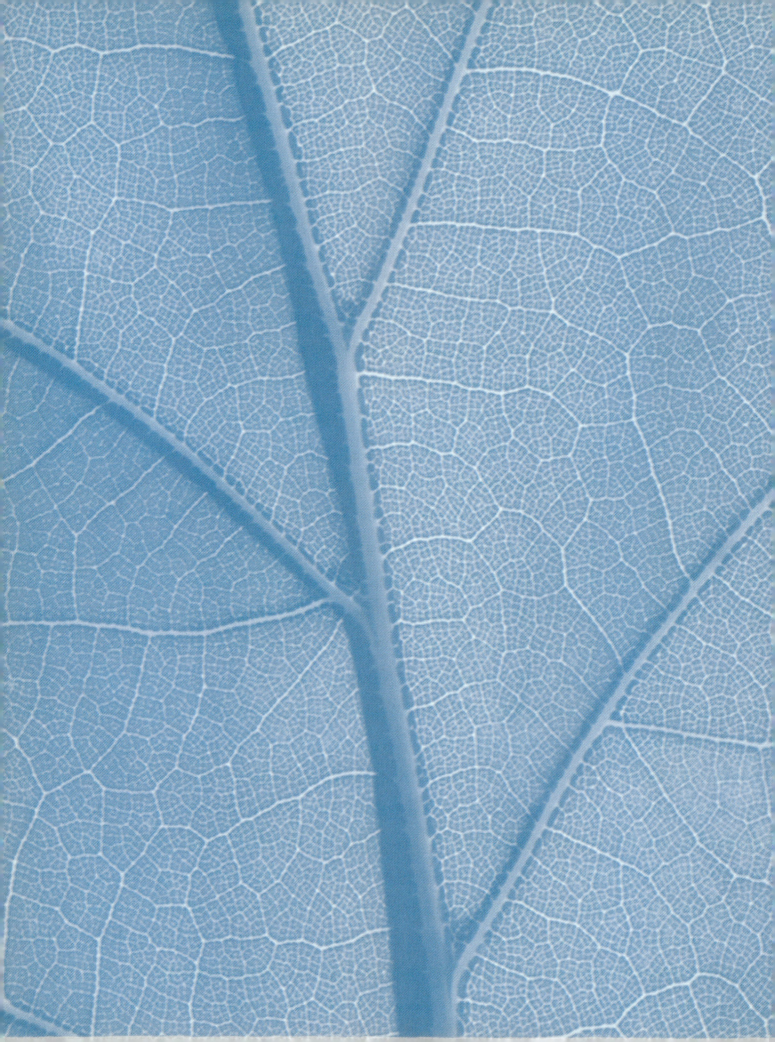

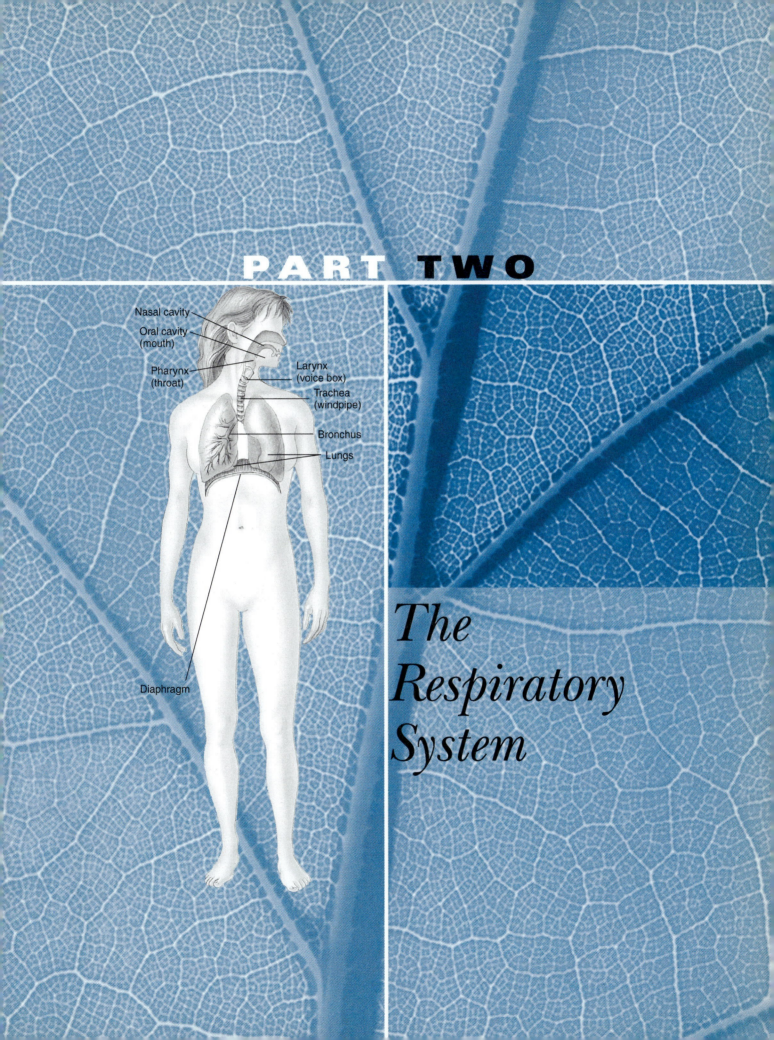

PART TWO

Nasal cavity

Oral cavity (mouth)

Pharynx (throat)

Larynx (voice box)

Trachea (windpipe)

Bronchus

Lungs

Diaphragm

The Respiratory System

Sara and Mary

GENDER

F

AGE

2 months old

SETTING

- Hospital

ETHNICITY

- White American

CULTURAL CONSIDERATIONS

PREEXISTING CONDITIONS

- Preterm birth

COEXISTING CONDITION

SIGNIFICANT HISTORY

COMMUNICATION

DISABILITY

SOCIOECONOMIC

SPIRITUAL

PHARMACOLOGIC

- Acetaminophen (Tylenol)
- Erythromycin lactobionate (Erythrocin IV)

PSYCHOSOCIAL

- Maternal anxiety
- Husband is out of town

LEGAL

ETHICAL

ALTERNATIVE THERAPY

PRIORITIZATION

- Yes

DELEGATION

- Yes

THE RESPIRATORY SYSTEM

Level of difficulty: Easy

Overview: This case requires knowledge of communicable disease, increased risk of infection secondary to preterm birth, intravenous therapy, as well as mother–child attachment relationship.

Client Profile

Sara and **Mary** are 2-month-old twins born at 35 weeks' gestation and weighing 2,272 g (81.1 oz) and 2,300 g (82.1 oz), respectively. They remained hospitalized for 4 weeks to gain weight and were discharged to home weighing 2,600 g (92.8 oz). They are scheduled to see the health care provider to begin their immunizations at 10 weeks of age. The twins' mother has taken an extended maternity leave to remain home with the twins until they are 4 months old.

Case Study

The twins' mother, Fran, noted that both infants, 9 weeks of age, had runny noses when she picked them up from daycare. The twins' father left at 5:00 A.M. for a 5-day business trip and at 6:00 A.M., Fran heard them both coughing. Their coughs sounded dry; however, when she checked them, they both had runny noses and felt warm to the touch. She took their temperatures; Sara's was 37.8° C (100° F) and Mary's was 38° C (100.4° F). She administered 15 mg/kg of acetaminophen. This lowered their temperatures to 37.4° C (99.3° F) and 37.5° C (99.25° F), respectively; however, they continued to cough. Three hours later, both girls began exhibiting a high-pitched, whooping sound when inhaling during their coughing attacks. When Fran noted the girls experienced brief apneic periods during their coughing spells and appeared "bluish" in color, she phoned her pediatrician and was told to go to the nearest emergency department. The girls were admitted to the pediatric nursing unit with a diagnosis of "rule out pertussis." Sara's leukocyte count is 31,000 cells/mm^3 and Fran's count is 32,300 cells/mm^3 on admission. Nasal and throat cultures and serology tests are pending. Intravenous access devices are placed and intravenous fluids of D_5W with .225% sodium chloride is initiated at 20 mL/hour. Their oxygen saturations are continuously monitored using pulse oximetry and each is started on 0.5 L of oxygen per nasal cannula in response to oxygen saturation readings of 94% for Sara and 92% for Mary. Arterial blood gases are drawn from each infant with the following results: For Sara: pH, 7.35; PCO_2, 35 mm Hg; PO_2, 90 mm Hg; oxygen saturation, 95%; and HCO_3, 22 mEq/L. For Mary: pH, 7.37; PCO_2, 37 mm Hg; PO_2, 85 mm Hg; oxygen saturation, 92%; and HCO_3, 23 mEq/L. On admission Sara weighs 2.9 kg (6 lb, 8 oz) and Mary weighs 3.2 kg (7 lb).

Questions

1. Which child should be seen by the nurse first and why?

2. Discuss pertussis and how it can be prevented.

3. What conclusions can you draw about the clinical manifestations and leukocyte counts of the twins?

4. Discuss the leukocyte results for the twins compared to normal values for these infants.

5. What is the significance of Sara and Mary's arterial blood gas results?

6. Explain the rationale for prescribing intravenous fluids for Sara and Mary.

7. Should the twins be placed on respiratory isolation to protect the nursing staff? Explain your answer.

8. Identify complications associated with pertussis that Sara and Mary are at risk for developing.

9. Identify the priority nursing diagnosis for Sara and Mary and appropriate nursing interventions.

10. The twins' mother is very quiet and appears on the verge of crying. She states, "It's all my fault and now I'm being punished. I shouldn't have worked during my pregnancy, but we couldn't afford for me to quit work, and then after the twins came home, I had to go back to work and leave them in daycare because my maternity leave had run out." How can you intervene to assist Fran?

11. The twins are prescribed erythromycin lactobionate 13 mg IV every 6 hours. Discuss why this agent is prescribed and if the prescribed dose is safe for Sara and Mary.

12. The twins respond favorably to treatment, and following a week of hospitalization their health care provider discharges them to home. Fran and her husband Jack are preparing for discharge. Discuss appropriate discharge instructions for this family.

Caleb

GENDER	**SOCIOECONOMIC**
M	
AGE	**SPIRITUAL**
6	
SETTING	**PHARMACOLOGIC**
■ Hospital	■ Atropine Sulfate
ETHNICITY	**PSYCHOSOCIAL**
■ Black American	■ Anxiety
CULTURAL CONSIDERATIONS	**LEGAL**
PREEXISTING CONDITIONS	**ETHICAL**
COEXISTING CONDITIONS	**ALTERNATIVE THERAPY**
SIGNIFICANT HISTORY	**PRIORITIZATION**
	■ Yes
COMMUNICATION	**DELEGATION**
	■ Yes
DISABILITY	

MODERATE

THE RESPIRATORY SYSTEM

Level of difficulty: Moderate

Overview: This case requires knowledge of growth and development and its impact on accidental injuries, normal respiratory function, cardiopulmonary resuscitation, mechanical ventilation, intravenous fluid therapy, as well as empathy for parental feelings/expressions of guilt.

Client Profile

Caleb is a 6-year-old boy in first grade. He lives with his mother and father and two siblings, a brother Tyler (8 years old) and a 10 year-old sister, Cherice. Caleb and his family are visiting his grandparents on their 40-acre farm in Minnesota for Thanksgiving. Caleb is an adventurous child who loves being active outdoors and enjoys swimming, fishing, soccer, and school activities.

Case Study

Mrs. Jones was inside the house helping her mother prepare the Thanksgiving dinner, and family were to arrive in 2 hours for the celebration. Mr. Jones was in the garage working on his mother-in-law's vehicle when Tyler came running to the house screaming that Caleb had fallen into the pond while they were fishing. Tyler said he had pulled him out but Caleb wasn't breathing. His father told Tyler to run into the house, call 911, and tell his mother what had happened. Mr. Jones ran to the pond and found Caleb lying face down on the pond bank. He turned Caleb over and confirmed that he was barely breathing. He covered Caleb with his coat, began calling for help, and remained with Caleb. After approximately 10 minutes, paramedics arrived and assessed Caleb. He had stopped breathing "about 5 minutes ago" according to his father. Caleb had a weak, but present pulse of 40 beats/minute. The paramedics performed abdominal thrusts and Caleb began coughing weakly, but remained unconscious. Oxygen was started at 100% per face mask and an intravenous access established. Lactated Ringer's intravenous solution was initiated while Caleb was transported to the local trauma center, where he was treated in the emergency department for immersion syndrome.

In the emergency department, Caleb's arterial blood gases were drawn and a pulse oximetry sensor was attached. The nurse performed a client history by talking to his parents. According to Mrs. Jones Caleb weighed 24.9 kg (55 lb) and was 1.3 m (4 ft, 2 in.) tall at his routine appointment with his pediatrician last week. His weight is confirmed, he is placed on a cardiorespiratory monitor, and atropine sulfate 0.5 mg intravenous is administered. His oxygen saturation was 80% and he is covered with warmed blankets. His vital signs on admission are: pulse, 45 beats/minute; respiratory rate, apneic; blood pressure, 50/30; and body temperature, 32.6° C (90.7° F). His arterial blood gas values are: pH, 7.29; $PaCO_3$, 50 mm Hg; PaO_2, 70 mm Hg; oxygen saturation, 75%; HCO_3, 24 mEq/L. Caleb is intubated and transferred to the pediatric intensive care unit, where mechanical ventilation is established.

Questions

1. What interpretations can you make based on Caleb's arterial blood gas results?

2. Discuss the factors that placed Caleb at risk for near drowning.

3. What other diagnostic test would be appropriate for the health care provider to prescribe for Caleb?

4. Explain the dive reflex and discuss whether this may have occurred in Caleb's case.

5. Discuss the intravenous fluids prescribed for Caleb including the rationale for their use in his case.

6. Caleb is placed on time-cycled positive pressure continuous mandatory ventilation. Discuss why this time-cycled positive pressure ventilation was chosen

by comparing it to the other types of positive pressure ventilation.

7. Discuss the difference between continuous mandatory ventilation and other types of mechanical ventilation modes.

8. Identify three priority nursing diagnoses for Caleb and how endotracheal intubation and mechanical ventilation can assist with these problems.

9. Caleb's father expresses to you that he feels "so guilty about Caleb and I shouldn't have let them go fishing alone." How do you respond to Mr. Jones?

10. After 14 days of hospitalization, Caleb recovers completely and is preparing for discharge. What should you include/stress in your discharge teaching?

Cara

GENDER	**SOCIOECONOMIC**
F	■ Middle class
AGE	**SPIRITUAL**
9 months old	
SETTING	**PHARMACOLOGIC**
■ Hospital	■ Metoclopramide (Maxolon)
ETHNICITY	■ Albuterol (Proventil)
■ White American	■ Ipratropium (Atrovent)
	■ Cefazolin Sodium (Ancef)
CULTURAL CONSIDERATIONS	**PSYCHOSOCIAL**
PREEXISTING CONDITIONS	**LEGAL**
■ Preterm birth	
COEXISTING CONDITIONS	**ETHICAL**
SIGNIFICANT HISTORY	**ALTERNATIVE THERAPY**
COMMUNICATION	**PRIORITIZATION**
DISABILITY	**DELEGATION**
	■ Health care team

MODERATE

THE RESPIRATORY SYSTEM

Level of difficulty: Moderate

Overview: This case requires knowledge of bronchopulmonary dysplasia, tracheostomy care and suctioning, growth and development, as well as an understanding of the client's background and personal situation.

Client Profile

Cara is a 9-month-old infant who was delivered by Cesarean section at 25 weeks' gestation secondary to premature rupture of the amniotic membranes. She weighed 1.1 kg (2.5 lb) at birth and required intubation and mechanical ventilation after birth. During her first month of life she required reintubation with each of three attempts to wean her from the ventilator. At 5 months of age, Cara was weaned from the ventilator, but still requires 38% oxygen by tracheostomy collar to maintain her oxygen saturation >92%. Currently, she weighs 4.9 kg (10.8 lb) and receives gastrostomy feedings of 80 mL of Neocate, 24-calorie formula, every 4 hours as a result of severe gastroesophageal reflux (GER). Prior to her daytime feedings, Cara receives metoclopramide 0.5 mg per gastric tube. The feedings are infused over 2 hours each, using a volumetric pump to prevent regurgitation. She requires tracheostomy suctioning every 2 hours for thick yellow-white mucous. She is receiving respiratory therapy with albuterol inhaler every 4 hours and Atrovent, (ipratropium) one puff every 8 hours. She also receives an iron supplement. During her hospital stay, Cara experienced two streptococcal pneumonia respiratory infections and required antibiotic therapy to resolve them. At 7 months of age Cara was discharged from the hospital with a diagnosis of bronchopulmonary dysplasia (BPD) into the care of her parents, Carolyn and Josh. Also at home is her 4-year-old brother Alex, who attends preschool three mornings a week.

Case Study

Cara was brought to the hospital yesterday after being seen by her pulmonary specialist at his office following her mother's call that Cara began experiencing respiratory distress at home. Her mother remains with her at the hospital and her father and brother visit every evening. The nurse from the day shift reported that Carolyn is very involved in her daughter's care, insisting on performing her morning care as well at her gastrostomy tube feedings and tracheostomy care and suctioning. The nurse observed Carolyn's care and found it followed appropriate procedures and protocols, but Carolyn is appearing very tired. She leaves only long enough to get a cup of coffee and a snack twice a day. She asks appropriate questions about her daughter's condition and spends all day holding and caring for her.

Questions

1. Discuss your impressions about the above situation.

2. What is the purpose of Cara being prescribed metoclopramide, and is her current dose safe?

3. What additional data would provide a better understanding of Cara's current condition?

4. Discuss the pathophysiology of BPD.

5. Is there a relationship between Cara's BPD and her GER?

6. Discuss why Cara requires gastrostomy feedings and the formula she is receiving.

7. What risk factors does Cara have for developing a respiratory infection?

8. Considering the client's compromised respiratory status, what precautions should be taken when suctioning her tracheostomy?

9. Your assessment of Cara's growth and development reveals that she responds to her mother's voice by turning toward the sound and tracking as her mother speaks; she rolls from her back to her side with no evidence of head lag; she is unable to sit without support and does not verbalize;

her palmar grasp has disappeared; and she is able to demonstrate a pincer grasp. She is unable to crawl, but moves herself in the crib on her stomach. How does Cara compare to other infants her age?

10. Following a chest x-ray and culture, Cara was diagnosed with a streptococcal pneumonia and prescribed cefazolin sodium 200 mg IV every 8 hours. Why is Cara prescribed this agent?

11. Would you question the dosage of cefazolin sodium prescribed? Why or why not?

12. How would you respond to Carolyn's fatigue?

13. Would a multidisciplinary health care team conference be appropriate for Cara and her family?

Erin

GENDER	**SOCIOECONOMIC**
F	
AGE	**SPIRITUAL**
8	
SETTING	**PHARMACOLOGIC**
■ Hospital	■ Ceftazidime (Tazicef)
ETHNICITY	■ Gentamicin (Garamycin)
	■ Vancomycin (Vancocin)
■ White American	**PSYCHOSOCIAL**
CULTURAL CONSIDERATIONS	■ Anxiety
	LEGAL
PREEXISTING CONDITIONS	
■ Cystic fibrosis	**ETHICAL**
COEXISTING CONDITIONS	
	ALTERNATIVE THERAPY
SIGNIFICANT HISTORY	
	PRIORITIZATION
COMMUNICATION	■ Yes
	DELEGATION
DISABILITY	■ Yes
■ Chronic disease	

THE RESPIRATORY SYSTEM

Level of difficulty: Difficult

Overview: This case requires knowledge of cystic fibrosis, growth and development, as well as understanding of the client's background, personal situation, and parent–child relationship.

DIFFICULT

Client Profile

Erin is an 8-year-old girl who lives with her parents and two younger sisters, Rachel, who is 5 years old, and Samantha, who is 2 years old. They live in a Midwestern community where Erin's father is a bank manager and her mother is a part-time investment broker who works from home, which allows her to stay at home with the children. Both of Erin's parents are very attentive to the children and are very knowledgeable about Erin's cystic fibrosis, which was diagnosed when Erin was 3 months old. Neither of her sisters has the disease. Erin takes pancreatic enzymes with each meal and snack (six doses per day) and she performs breathing exercises twice a day. Her mother performs postural drainage 1 hour prior to breakfast, again when Erin returns from school in the afternoon, and finally each evening prior to Erin's going to bed.

Case Study

During late spring Erin's breathing has become increasingly congested over the past week and her parents suspect that she has developed a respiratory infection when she becomes febrile with a temperature of 37.9° C (100.2° F). They phone her pediatrician, who recommends that she be admitted to the children's hospital 20 miles away. The pediatrician calls the hospital and informs the chief respiratory resident physician of Erin's history, chief complaints at present, and impending arrival. Sputum cultures, complete blood count, serum electrolyte panel, chest x-ray, and pulmonary function diagnostics are prescribed. Erin's last admission for pulmonary clean-out was 6 months ago. Erin is admitted and her diagnostic results include hemoglobin, 18 g/dL; hematocrit, 51%; white blood cell count, 15,000 cells/mm³; platelets, 250,000 cells/mm³; red blood cell count, 5.1 million cells/mm³; serum glucose, 130 mg/dL; potassium, 4.0 mmol/L; sodium, 130 mmol/L; chloride, 90 mmol/L; blood urea nitrogen (BUN), 26 mg/dL; and creatinine, 0.7 mg/dL. Her chest x-ray shows consolidation in her right lower and middle lobes, and her oxygen saturation is 89%. Erin's pulmonary function is determined to be 45% and as you are compiling Erin's history, her mother tells you that Erin has been on the lung transplant list for 9 months. Erin weighs 44 lb on admission.

Questions

1. Discuss your impressions about Erin's diagnostic values.

2. Discuss what risks Erin has for developing a pulmonary infection.

3. What pertinent information is missing?

4. Identify the common microorganisms that cause respiratory infections in a child with cystic fibrosis.

5. What is the relationship between Erin's condition and her oxygen saturation level?

6. The health care provider prescribes ceftazidime 1 g IV every 8 hours; gentamicin 50 mg IV every 8 hours; and vancomycin 265 mg IV every 8 hours. Discuss why these drugs are prescribed for Erin.

7. Discuss the safety and efficacy of the doses of the antimicrobial agents prescribed for Erin.

8. What are the criteria established for lung transplant candidates?

9. Erin's condition worsens, and when no cadaver lungs are available, Erin's mother states that she wants to donate part or all of one of her lungs to Erin. After testing her mother for compatibility, the surgeon decides to proceed with the transplant the following day. Identify the priority client problems for Erin following the transplant.

10. Discuss the common immunosuppressant agents used to prevent organ rejection.

11. Erin receives a single lung transplant. Discuss what the risks are for her cystic fibrosis recurring in her transplant lung.

12. Erin and her mother recover from the surgery. Discuss the teaching priorities you will address with Erin and her parents prior to Erin's discharge.

13. What are the current statistics for successful lung transplants?

Anna

GENDER

F

AGE

4

SETTING

- Hospital

ETHNICITY

- White American

CULTURAL CONSIDERATIONS

PREEXISTING CONDITIONS

- Autism

COEXISTING CONDITIONS

SIGNIFICANT HISTORY

COMMUNICATION

- Child is nonverbal

DISABILITY

SOCIOECONOMIC

SPIRITUAL

PHARMACOLOGIC

PSYCHOSOCIAL

- Anxiety
- Caregiver stress

LEGAL

ETHICAL

ALTERNATIVE THERAPY

- Vitamins

PRIORITIZATION

- Yes

DELEGATION

- Yes

THE RESPIRATORY SYSTEM

Level of difficulty: Moderate

Overview: This case requires knowledge of autism, the role of alternative therapy in this child's care, tonsillitis, growth and development, as well as an understanding of the client's background, personal situation, and parent–child relationship.

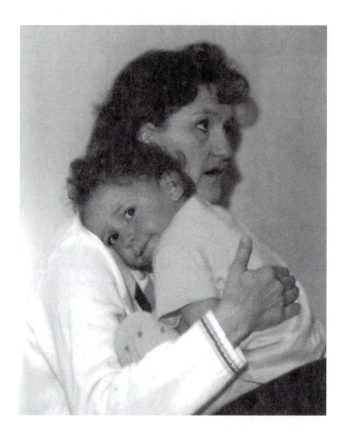

Client Profile

Anna is a 4-year-old autistic preschooler who lives at home with her parents and three older siblings. Anna is nonverbal, although she intermittently cries out while playing and can be disruptive at home. She attends a Head Start educational program in town and, according to her teacher, her behavior at school has gradually become less disruptive. Over the past year, she has experienced three episodes of tonsillitis. With each episode she was treated with antibiotics that seemed to effectively treat the problem until the next episode occurred. Following treatment for her last episode a month ago, her pediatrician recommended a tonsillectomy. Her parents are quite anxious at the thought of Anna having surgery and being hospitalized. The surgery is scheduled for the following week.

Case Study

During her preoperative visit Anna is very quiet and clings to her mother. Her parents speak and understand sufficient English to communicate with the nurse. They express their concerns about Anna having surgery and state that they have given her daily vitamins since she was just a baby to help prevent her from getting "these kinds of infections." Further, they have avoided talking about Anna's situation at home because they don't want to increase the child's anxiety. They state she would be very afraid if surrounded by strangers. They explain to the nurse that Anna has autism and express their concerns about the child's response to hospitalization because her behavior worsens when she is in an unfamiliar environment. Anna weighs 35 lb.

Questions

1. What is autism and what is its incidence and etiology?

2. Discuss the potential impact Anna's autism may have on her hospital experience.

3. Discuss the parents' comment about giving Anna vitamins to prevent "these kinds of infections."

4. How can the nurse interact to address the family's anxiety?

5. Discuss the incidence and causes of tonsillitis.

6. What diagnostic studies should be performed prior to Anna's surgery?

7. Anna is admitted to the same-day surgical unit and is accompanied by her parents. When approached, her parents verbalize that Anna is afraid that the "people are going to hurt her." How should the nurse respond to Anna and her parents?

8. What are the nursing priorities for Anna's postoperative care?

9. Discuss the appropriate priority nursing interventions for Anna.

10. Anna refuses to take fluids following her surgery and her urine output has decreased. She is then transferred to the pediatric surgical unit for an overnight stay. What is the rationale for this action? What is the expected urine output for Anna, who weighs 15.9 kg (35 lb)?

11. Anna cries and becomes withdrawn when visiting hours on the unit are over as her parents prepare to go home to check on their other children. Discuss Anna's reaction, relating it to her growth and development and the impact hospitalization has on a child Anna's age.

12. What could the nurse do to decrease Anna's anxiety and minimize the stressors of hospitalization?

13. Anna's mother spends the night with her, and the following morning Anna is drinking and her urine output is within normal limits so she is to be discharged. Discuss the discharge teaching for Anna and her parents.

CASE STUDY 6

Dwight

GENDER

M

AGE

4

SETTING

- Hospital

ETHNICITY

- White American

CULTURAL CONSIDERATIONS

PREEXISTING CONDITIONS

- Recurrent otitis media

COEXISTING CONDITIONS

SIGNIFICANT HISTORY

COMMUNICATION

DISABILITY

SOCIOECONOMIC

SPIRITUAL

PHARMACOLOGIC

- EMLA

PSYCHOSOCIAL

- Client anxiety and fear

LEGAL

- Informed consent

ETHICAL

ALTERNATIVE THERAPY

PRIORITIZATION

- Yes

DELEGATION

THE RESPIRATORY SYSTEM

Level of difficulty: Easy

Overview: This case requires knowledge of surgical preparation, growth and development, as well as an understanding of the client's background, personal situation, and family–child relationship.

171

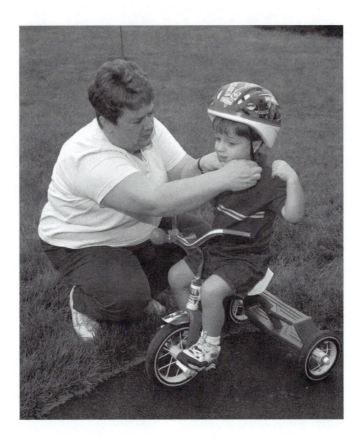

Client Profile   **Dwight** is a 4-year-old who lives with his parents and 18-month-old sister. Dwight's parents decided to send him to preschool when he turned 3 years old to provide him with contact and interactions with other preschoolers. Dwight loves going to "school"; however, over the past year Dwight has experienced recurrent episodes of otitis media (OM) secondary to respiratory infections. Following his last episode of OM, his pediatrician suggested to his parents that Dwight should have "tubes put in his ears."

Case Study   On a follow-up visit, Dwight's parents discuss the surgery and decide to have it performed. Dwight's surgery is scheduled in 5 days.

Questions

1. Discuss who is responsible for preparing Dwight psychosocially for his hospitalization and surgery.

2. When should the preoperative teaching begin for Dwight and what topics should be addressed?

3. Dwight is admitted to the hospital in the morning and his surgery is scheduled for 2:00 P.M. Discuss the stressors for the preschooler who is hospitalized in terms of their priority.

4. What are the priorities of care for Dwight on admission?

5. Describe therapeutic nursing interventions that can lessen Dwight's stressors.

6. The nurse discusses with Dwight's parents that he needs to have an intravenous access initiated. Dwight is visibly upset and begins to cry, telling his mother, "Don't let them hurt me!!" What measures should the nurse take prior to performing Dwight's venipuncture?

7. Discuss the difference between the parents' informed consent and Dwight's assent for surgery.

8. Discuss the importance of including Dwight in the surgical preparation process.

9. How can a health care facility address a child's separation anxiety as the child is being transferred to the preoperative hold area and later in the PICU following surgery?

10. Discuss the nursing priorities of care for Dwight following his surgical procedure.

CASE STUDY 7

Helen

GENDER

F

AGE

10 months old

SETTING

- Clinic

ETHNICITY

- White American

CULTURAL CONSIDERATIONS

PREEXISTING CONDITIONS

COEXISTING CONDITIONS

SIGNIFICANT HISTORY

COMMUNICATION

DISABILITY

SOCIOECONOMIC

- Middle class

SPIRITUAL

PHARMACOLOGIC

- Amoxicillin (Amoxil)
- Amoxicillin and clavulanate potassium (Augmentin)

PSYCHOSOCIAL

- Growth and development

LEGAL

ETHICAL

ALTERNATIVE THERAPY

PRIORITIZATION

DELEGATION

MODERATE

THE RESPIRATORY SYSTEM

Level of difficulty: Moderate

Overview: This case requires knowledge of tobacco addiction, otitis media, growth and development, as well as an understanding of the client's background, personal situation, and family relationship.

Client Profile

Helen is a 10-month-old girl who lives with her parents and two siblings. Her mother has just returned to work after being at home for 3 years as a "stay-at-home mom." For financial reasons, her mother has decided to resume her career as a nurse. Helen, her 2-year-old brother Hunter, and 3-year-old sister Emily are now attending a daycare center near their home while their parents are at work. All were breastfed and weaned to the bottle at 7 months of age. Helen is now being bottlefed. The family lives in a middle-class neighborhood, and the father is a heavy smoker, having smoked cigarettes for 10 years.

Case Study

Last week Helen developed an upper respiratory infection after being exposed to an infected child at the daycare center. Five days later her mother took her to the pediatrician's office for fever of 38.3° C (101° F), fussiness, decreased appetite, pulling on her right ear, and crying. During the visit the nurse practitioner examines Helen and on otoscopic exam notes that Helen's right tympanic membrane is bulging, red, and opaque with a small amount of purulent drainage in the ear canal. Helen weighs 19.8 lb and is placed on amoxicillin 250 mg t.i.d. for 10 days. Nine days into the regimen of amoxicillin, Helen's mother brings her back to the pediatrician's office with symptoms similar to those that began 2 days ago, including crying, diarrhea, vomiting, and pulling at her right ear. This morning Helen was experiencing a fever of 38.3° C (101° F) that prompted her mother to return to the office. Helen is prescribed Augmentin (amoxicillin and clavulanate potassium) 400 mg q8h in a suspension containing 400 mg/5 mL for 10 days.

Questions

1. Discuss your impressions about the above situation.

2. What risk factors does Helen have for developing acute otitis media (OM)?

3. Discuss the difference between acute OM and chronic OM.

4. Discuss the relationship between Helen's recent enrollment in daycare and her condition.

5. What is the relationship between upper respiratory infections and the development of OM?

6. OM is the leading cause of what sensory deficit? Discuss this process.

7. How does passive cigarette smoke increase Helen's risk for OM?

8. Discuss how you could approach Helen's father about his smoking and the risks it poses to his family.

9. Discuss the relationship between amoxicillin suspension and Augmentin (amoxicillin and clavulanate potassium), including the pediatrician's reasons for changing antibiotics before the course of amoxicillin was completed.

10. The safe dose of Augmentin (amoxicillin and clavulanate potassium) is 90 mg/kg per day. What is the safe range for Helen and is the prescribed dose safe for her?

11. Develop the priority nursing diagnoses that apply to Helen related to her OM.

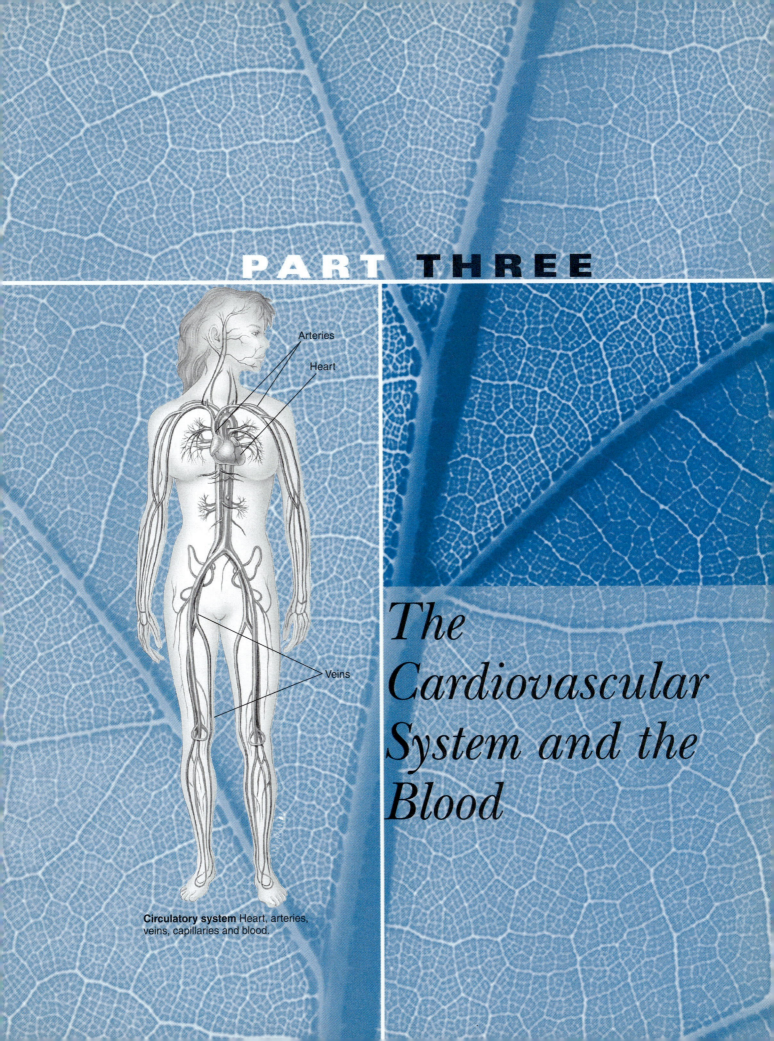

PART THREE

Arteries

Heart

Veins

Circulatory system Heart, arteries, veins, capillaries and blood.

The Cardiovascular System and the Blood

Nisha

GENDER

F

AGE

14

SETTING

- Hospital

ETHNICITY

- Black American

CULTURE CONSIDERATIONS

PREEXISTING CONDITIONS

COEXISTING CONDITIONS

- Sickle cell anemia

SIGNIFICANT HISTORY

COMMUNICATION

DISABILITY

SOCIOECONOMIC

SPIRITUAL

PHARMACOLOGIC

- Morphine sulfate (Duramorph)
- Acetaminophen (Tylenol)

PSYCHOSOCIAL

- Client anxiety
- Parent anxiety

LEGAL

ETHICAL

ALTERNATIVE THERAPY

PRIORITIZATION

- Yes

DELEGATION

- Client teaching

THE CIRCULATORY SYSTEM

Level of difficulty: Easy

Overview: This case requires knowledge of sickle cell disease, growth and development, as well as an understanding of the client's background, and personal situation, and mother–child attachment relationship.

Client Profile

Nisha is a 14-year-old with sickle cell anemia. She lives with her mother and grandmother in a rural neighborhood. Nisha has experienced several "sickle cell crises," however, they seem to have become more frequent since she became an adolescent. Nisha is enjoying her summer break from school. She is active in softball and enjoys shopping with her girlfriends.

Case Study

Nisha's mother brings her to the hematology clinic at the hospital with complaints of severe generalized pain following a softball game in which she pitched seven innings. She is admitted to the medical pediatric unit. Her vital signs are: temperature, 37.6° C (99.7° F); pulse 110 beats/minute; respiration, 30 breaths/minute; and blood pressure, 96/70. She weighs 110 lb. Her complete blood count reveals: hemoglobin, 9 g/dL; hematocrit, 24%; white blood cell count, 12,000 cells/mm^3; and platelet count, 140,000 cells/mm^3. Her oxygen saturation is 89%.

Questions

1. Discuss your impressions of Nisha's clinical manifestations.

2. Discuss the pathophysiology of sickle cell anemia.

3. What causes sickle cell anemia and how common is it?

4. What is sickle cell crisis?

5. What other assessment data would be helpful for the nurse to have to prepare Nisha's care plan?

6. What are the priorities of care for Nisha on admission?

7. The health care provider prescribes the following for Nisha:

Vital signs q4h. Notify health care provider of temperature >38° C (100.4° F)

Regular diet

Strict bedrest

Complete blood count with differential in the morning

Urine for urinalysis (U/A) and culture and sensitivity (C/S)

Chest x-ray

IV fluids of 5% dextrose in water with .45% normal saline to infuse at 175 mL/hour

PCA morphine sulfate 1.5 mg continuous and 1 mg every 8 minutes, PCA dose

Acetaminophen 650 mg q4h PO for temperature >38° C (100.4° F)

Oxygen at 2 L per nasal cannula, titrating to maintain oxygen saturation >94%

Discuss these prescriptions and if the nurse should question any of them.

8. What nursing interventions would be appropriate in meeting Nisha's needs?

9. After 4 days of treatment, Nisha's intravenous fluids and medication are discontinued and her pain assessment reveals a pain level of 1/10. When the nurse enters Nisha's room, Nisha is sitting quietly in a chair at the bedside and seems sad. Discuss your impressions of Nisha's condition based on her level of growth and development.

10. Discuss the teaching priorities for Nisha before her discharge from the hospital after her crisis is resolved.

CASE STUDY 2

Brandon

GENDER

M

AGE

8

SETTING

- Clinic/hospital

ETHNICITY

- White American

CULTURE CONSIDERATIONS

PREEXISTING CONDITIONS

- Hemophilia A

COEXISTING CONDITIONS

- Hemophilia A

SIGNIFICANT HISTORY

COMMUNICATION

DISABILITY

SOCIOECONOMIC

- Middle class

SPIRITUAL

PHARMACOLOGIC

- Acetaminophen (Tylenol)

PSYCHOSOCIAL

- Parental and client anxiety

LEGAL

ETHICAL

ALTERNATIVE THERAPY

PRIORITIZATION

- Hourly assessments

DELEGATION

- Nursing assistant
- Yes

THE BLOOD

Level of difficulty: Moderate

Overview: This case requires knowledge of hemophilia, growth and development, as well as an understanding of the client's background, personal situation, and parent–client relationship.

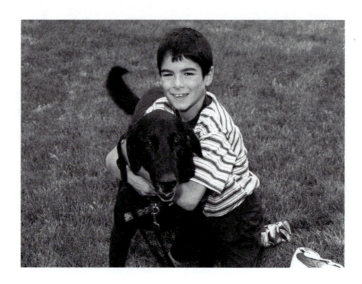

Client Profile

Brandon is an 8-year-old with a history of hemophilia A, diagnosed when he was 13 months old. He lives with his parents and 10-year-old and 6-year-old sisters. He attends the local grade school with his sisters and routinely receives factor replacement at the hematology clinic. The family has adjusted well to Brandon's diagnosis although he has required hospitalization for hemarthrosis twice since he was a preschooler.

Case Study

Brandon experiences an abrasion and some contusions while playing on the play ground at school. It has been 6 months since his last factor replacement, and when the abrasions continue to bleed and the contusions increase in size, his parents take him to the clinic.

Questions

1. Discuss hemophilia and its incidence.

2. Discuss how factor replacement is administered in a clinic setting and the specific nursing responsibilities associated with factor replacement.

3. Discuss the risks of human immunodeficiency virus (HIV) and hepatitis transmission and transfusion reactions as a result of factor replacement.

4. For the past 2 months, Brandon has not had any other injuries; however, his mother notices that his right knee is slightly swollen and he is starting to limp when he walks. What is your impression of Brandon's current condition as it relates to his level of growth and development?

5. Brandon and his mother return to the hematology clinic and his health care provider determines that he should be admitted to the hospital. Why do you think Brandon's health care provider makes the decision to admit Brandon for treatment now?

6. What are the priorities of care for Brandon?

7. Brandon is admitted to the pediatric unit and prescribed the following:

   a. Draw serum factor VIII now

   b. Placed in 15 lb of traction

   c. Diet as tolerated

   d. Vital signs routine

   e. Establish peripheral intravenous access and medlock

   f. Uninalysis now

   g. Hemocult all stools

   h. Acetaminophen 325 mg PO every 4 hours as needed for pain

Discuss the above prescriptions. Would the nurse question any of them? What about Brandon's activity level?

8. Brandon has just been placed in traction at the shift change on the pediatric unit. His nurse should make what routine (hourly) assessments on Brandon?

9. The nurse is assigned a nursing assistant to work with her in providing care for her four pediatric clients. What aspects of Brandon's care can the nurse delegate to the nursing assistant?

10. Brandon's factor result is 20 mg/100 mL. Explain the significance of this result.

11. Brandon's mother, who remains at Brandon's bedside throughout his hospitalization, tells the nurse that Brandon is complaining of being "stiff" and " so bored." How should the nurse respond to Brandon and his mother?

12. After 2 weeks of hospitalization, Brandon is preparing to be discharged. Discuss the client and family teaching the nurse should perform prior to Brandon's discharge.

Ryan

GENDER

M

AGE

11 months old

SETTING

- Hospital

ETHNICITY

- White American

CULTURE CONSIDERATIONS

PREEXISTING CONDITIONS

COEXISTING CONDITIONS

- Atrial septal defect

SIGNIFICANT HISTORY

COMMUNICATION

DISABILITY

- Down syndrome

SOCIOECONOMIC

SPIRITUAL

PHARMACOLOGIC

- Digoxin (Lanoxin)
- Furosemide (Lasix)

PSYCHOSOCIAL

- Parental anxiety

LEGAL

ETHICAL

ALTERNATIVE THERAPY

PRIORITIZATION

- Yes

DELEGATION

- Client teaching

DIFFICULT

THE CARDIOVASCULAR SYSTEM

Level of difficulty: Difficult

Overview: This case requires knowledge of normal and abnormal heart function; understanding of the client's background, personal situation, and parent–child relationship; and management of client pain.

Client Profile

Ryan is an 11-month-old infant who was born with Down's syndrome and lives with his parents in a middle-class neighborhood. Ryan weighed 3.2 kg (7 lb) at birth and a heart murmur was heard. Ryan was breast fed for 4 months. His mother says that at the time, he became "disinterested" in the breastfeeding, but when she was able to get him to nurse, he would fall asleep after having nursed for only 5 minutes. Because he was not gaining weight appropriately, his pediatrician prescribed infant formula with iron and suggested that his mother begin feeding Ryan rice cereal twice a day. At 4 months of age Ryan was diagnosed with an atrial septal defect that has been monitored since the diagnosis. Ryan sits unsupported but, according to his mother, does not crawl or attempt to stand because "he gets out of breath when he tries to crawl so we bought a walker that he moves around in." Since he was 5 months old, Ryan has been receiving digoxin 200 μg and furosemide 10 mg every day.

Case Study

Ryan's parents bring Ryan in to see his cardiologist because he has been lethargic and has had diarrhea for the past 24 hours. When the nurse assesses Ryan, she finds he weighs 7 kg (15.4 lb) and his vital signs are:

Temperature: 36.5° C (97.7° F)

Pulse: 80 beats/minute

Respirations – 35 breaths/minute

His laboratory results are:

Potassium level: 2.9 mmol/L

Digoxin level: 2.5 ng/mL

Questions

1. Discuss the pathophysiology of atrial septal defect.

2. What is the incidence and etiology of this congenital heart defect?

3. What is the relationship between Ryan's current weight and his heart defect?

4. What other assessment data indicate the impact on Ryan's growth and development?

5. Discuss the rationale for the medication regimen for Ryan.

6. What is your impression of Ryan's assessment data at the cardiologist's office?

7. Ryan's cardiologist determines that Ryan's atrial septal defect should be surgically repaired. What preoperative assessment data is required prior to Ryan's surgery?

8. What are the priorities for Ryan's preoperative care?

9. Discuss the potential complications associated with open heart surgery performed on an infant.

10. Ryan's parents are very anxious about his surgery and expressing concern about what they are going to see when they get to visit him in the pediatric critical care unit after his surgery. How can the nurse intervene to help Ryan's parents prepare for their visit?

11. His parents express great concern about Ryan's pain management following surgery. They've heard that "some doctors don't think infants feel that much pain and what they do feel they don't remember." They have talked to Ryan's surgeon, who has reassured them that Ryan will be adequately medicated to control his pain after surgery. What should the nurse do in response to their concerns?

12. Ryan successfully undergoes open heart surgery to repair his atrial septal defect. Discuss the reason and purpose of the chest tubes placed in Ryan.

13. What are the nursing responsibilities associated with the care of Ryan's chest tubes?

14. What are the priorities of care for Ryan during his postoperative stay in the pediatric critical care unit?

15. Discuss nursing interventions to meet the goals of care for Ryan.

16. Ryan is transferred from the pediatric critical care unit to the pediatric surgical unit. Five days later his parents are preparing to take him home. Discuss the teaching priorities for Ryan's parents prior to his discharge.

Sean

GENDER	**SOCIOECONOMIC**
M	■ Middle class
AGE	**SPIRITUAL**
1 month old	
SETTING	**PHARMACOLOGIC**
■ Hospital	■ Antibiotics during pregnancy
ETHNICITY	**PSYCHOSOCIAL**
■ White American	■ Parental anxiety
CULTURE CONSIDERATIONS	**LEGAL**
PREEXISTING CONDITIONS	**ETHICAL**
COEXISTING CONDITIONS	**ALTERNATIVE THERAPY**
SIGNIFICANT HISTORY	**PRIORITIZATION**
	■ Yes
COMMUNICATION	**DELEGATION**
	■ Yes
DISABILITY	

THE CARDIOVASCULAR SYSTEM

Level of difficulty: Difficult

Overview: This case requires knowledge of organ transplantation, immunosuppressant therapy, growth and development, as well as parent–child attachment relationship.

DIFFICULT

Client Profile

Sean is the first child for John and Jenny, a 27-year-old couple who live in a suburb of a large city. Jenny's pregnancy was uneventful until the eighth month of Sean's gestation, when Jenny developed a severe respiratory infection that required 10 days of antibiotic therapy. At 40 weeks' gestation Sean was born weighing 3 kg (6 lb 8 oz) and was 47.5 cm (19 in.) long. Jenny planned to breast feed and had quit her part-time job to stay home with her baby. Sean's Apgar scores at 1 minute and 5 minutes were 4 and 6, respectively, so he was admitted to the neonatal intensive care unit.

Case Study

Sean is stabilized but unable to maintain his oxygen saturation >50% unless receiving 100% oxygen. This treatment sustains an 90% oxygen saturation. Following diagnostic evaluation, Sean is diagnosed with severe hypoplastic left heart syndrome (HLHS). When the pediatric cardiologist explains Sean's heart defect, she explains that she would like to place Sean on extra corporeal membrane oxygenator (ECMO) and keep him in the hospital until he is 1-month-old, if possible, and then perform surgery to repair his heart. After the surgeon leaves, Jenny says to the nurse, "I know this is my fault because of the antibiotics I took last month. I didn't mean to hurt my baby." She begins to cry as John attempts to comfort her.

Questions

1. Describe HLHS.

2. What is the appropriate response for the nurse concerning Sean's parents' feelings of guilt?

3. Discuss the clinical manifestations of HLHS.

4. How is HLHS diagnosed?

5. Discuss nursing interventions specific to the diagnostic tests Sean will undergo.

6. Describe the most commonly used surgical treatment for HLHS.

7. Sean undergoes unsuccessful reconstructive surgery for his HLHS and the decision is made that Sean needs a heart transplant. How common are heart transplants in children younger than 1 year of age?

8. Discuss the complications associated with heart transplants in children.

9. A donor for Sean was located and plans went into action for Sean to receive his transplant. Discuss the process of matching the donor heart prior to the transplantation into Sean.

10. The heart transplant procedure was successful. What is the standard of care to prevent rejection of Sean's transplanted heart?

11. Discuss the priorities of care for Sean following his heart transplant.

12. Discuss the priorities of teaching for Sean's parents during his hospitalization. When should the teaching begin? How can the nurse evaluate the effectiveness of the teaching?

Cassie

GENDER

F

AGE

9

SETTING

- Hospital

ETHNICITY

- Black American

CULTURE CONSIDERATIONS

PREEXISTING CONDITIONS

COEXISTING CONDITIONS

SIGNIFICANT HISTORY

COMMUNICATION

DISABILITY

SOCIOECONOMIC

- Middle class

SPIRITUAL

PHARMACOLOGIC

PSYCHOSOCIAL

- Mother died 6 years ago
- Parent anxiety
- Client anxiety
- Grieving

LEGAL

ETHICAL

- Do not resuscitate order

ALTERNATIVE THERAPY

PRIORITIZATION

- Yes

DELEGATION

- Client referrals

DIFFICULT

THE BLOOD

Level of difficulty: Difficult

Overview: This case requires knowledge and understanding of aplastic anemia, the grief response, additional care measures for the grieving family, as well as an understanding of the client's background, personal situation, and father–child relationship.

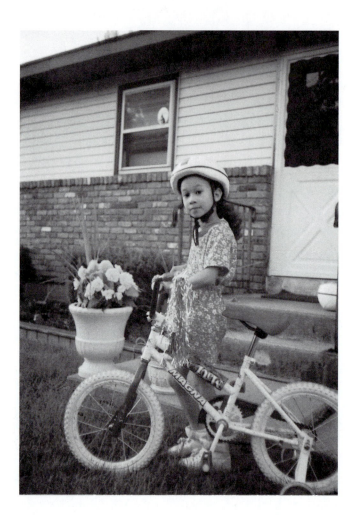

Client Profile

Cassie is a 9-year-old fourth grader who lives in a small community with her father, grandmother, and two older siblings. Cassie's mother died when Cassie was 3 years old and her father and grandmother are raising the children. They are very attentive to all of them, helping the children with their homework and attending their school activities. Cassie's father owns an automobile repair shop and her grandmother is active in the community. During the past 2 months, Cassie, who was always a healthy and active child, has become increasingly more fatigued; her appetite has become poor; and she is no longer interested in school, complaining each school day morning that she is too tired to go to school even though she sleeps 10 hours each night. Previously an A–B student, she is now doing poorly. Both her father and grandmother have noticed that Cassie is bruising easily, coughing frequently, and has a temperature. They are concerned about Cassie and her father makes an appointment with her pediatrician.

Case Study

After visiting her pediatrician, Cassie is admitted to the local hospital for tests to rule out aplastic anemia. Her admission vital signs are:

Temperature: 38° C (100.4° F)

Pulse: 120 beats/minute

Respirations: 30 breaths/minute

Blood pressure: 100/62

Cassie's admission complete blood count is:

Hemoglobin: 8 g/dL

Hematocrit: 25%

Erythrocyte count: 3.1 million/mm³

Platelet count: 80,000/mm³

White blood cell: 900 cells/mm³

Neutrophils: 630 cells/mm³

Lymphocytes: 180 cells/mm³

Monocytes: 63 cells/mm³

Eosinophils: 18 cells/mm³

Basophils: 9 cells/mm³

Questions

1. What other information would help you gain a fuller impression about Cassie's situation?

2. What is the significance of Cassie's lab values and vital signs?

3. Discuss the three types of aplastic anemia.

4. Discuss the incidence of and prognosis for aplastic anemia.

5. Identity the priorities of care for Cassie.

6. Discuss the treatment you anticipate for Cassie.

7. Discuss the nursing responsibilities prior to and during Cassie's blood products administration.

8. Cassie does not respond to treatment and after a bone marrow transplant fails, her condition worsens as her lab values decline. How can you respond to her father and grandmother when they ask if she is going to die?

9. Cassie's health care provider tells her father and grandmother that Cassie's condition is terminal. They say they want to take her home to die, but the health care provider is reluctant. How might you feel in a similar situation if Cassie was your child?

10. Cassie's father and grandmother prepare to take Cassie home. What referrals might benefit this family?

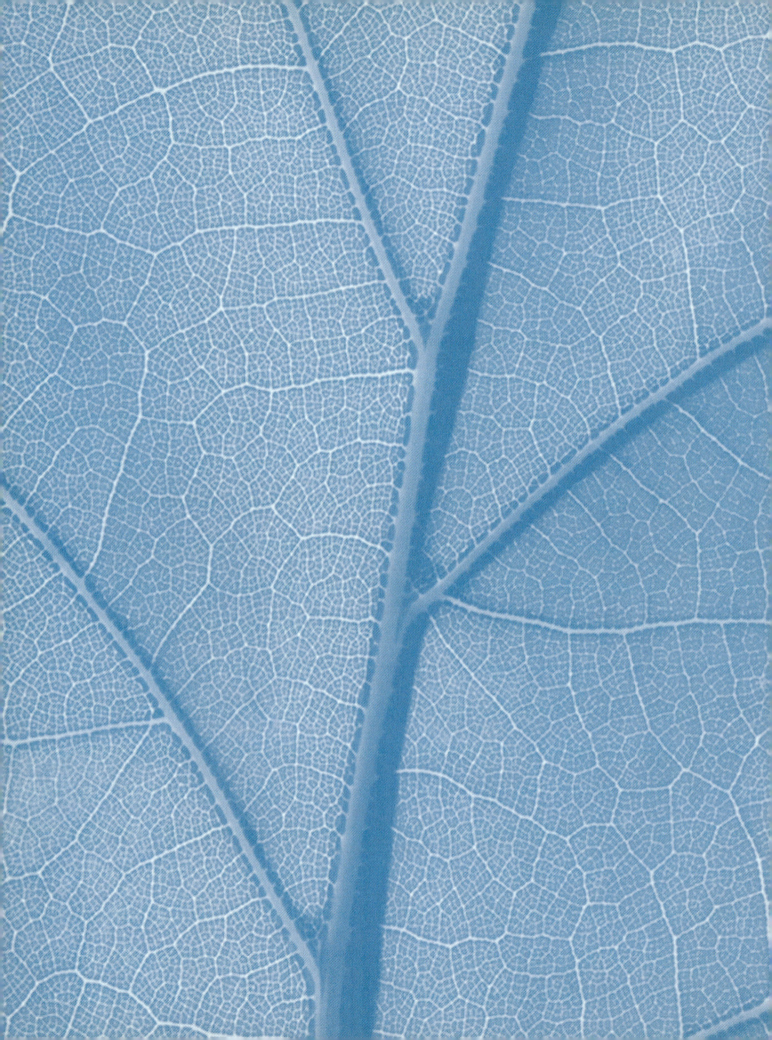

Blood pressure: 100/62

Cassie's admission complete blood count is:

Hemoglobin: 8 g/dL

Hematocrit: 25%

Erythrocyte count: 3.1 million/mm^3

Platelet count: 80,000/mm^3

White blood cell: 900 cells/mm^3

Neutrophils: 630 cells/mm^3

Lymphocytes: 180 cells/mm^3

Monocytes: 63 cells/mm^3

Eosinophils: 18 cells/mm^3

Basophils: 9 cells/mm^3

Questions

1. What other information would help you gain a fuller impression about Cassie's situation?

2. What is the significance of Cassie's lab values and vital signs?

3. Discuss the three types of aplastic anemia.

4. Discuss the incidence of and prognosis for aplastic anemia.

5. Identity the priorities of care for Cassie.

6. Discuss the treatment you anticipate for Cassie.

7. Discuss the nursing responsibilities prior to and during Cassie's blood products administration.

8. Cassie does not respond to treatment and after a bone marrow transplant fails, her condition worsens as her lab values decline. How can you respond to her father and grandmother when they ask if she is going to die?

9. Cassie's health care provider tells her father and grandmother that Cassie's condition is terminal. They say they want to take her home to die, but the health care provider is reluctant. How might you feel in a similar situation if Cassie was your child?

10. Cassie's father and grandmother prepare to take Cassie home. What referrals might benefit this family?

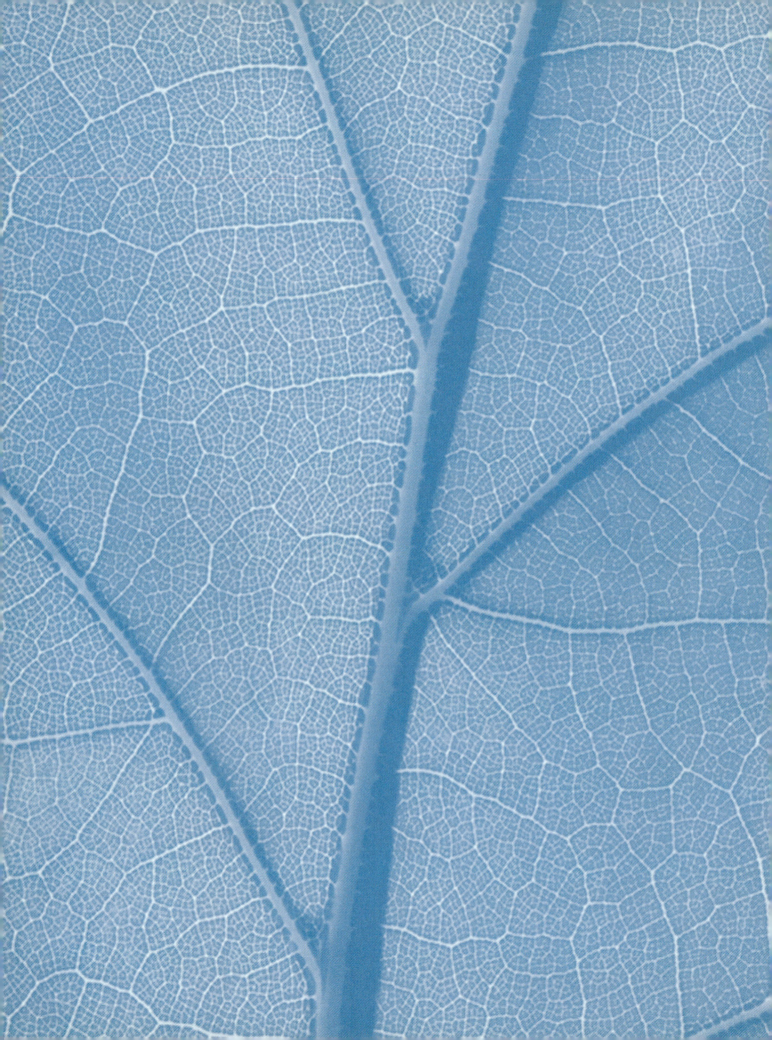

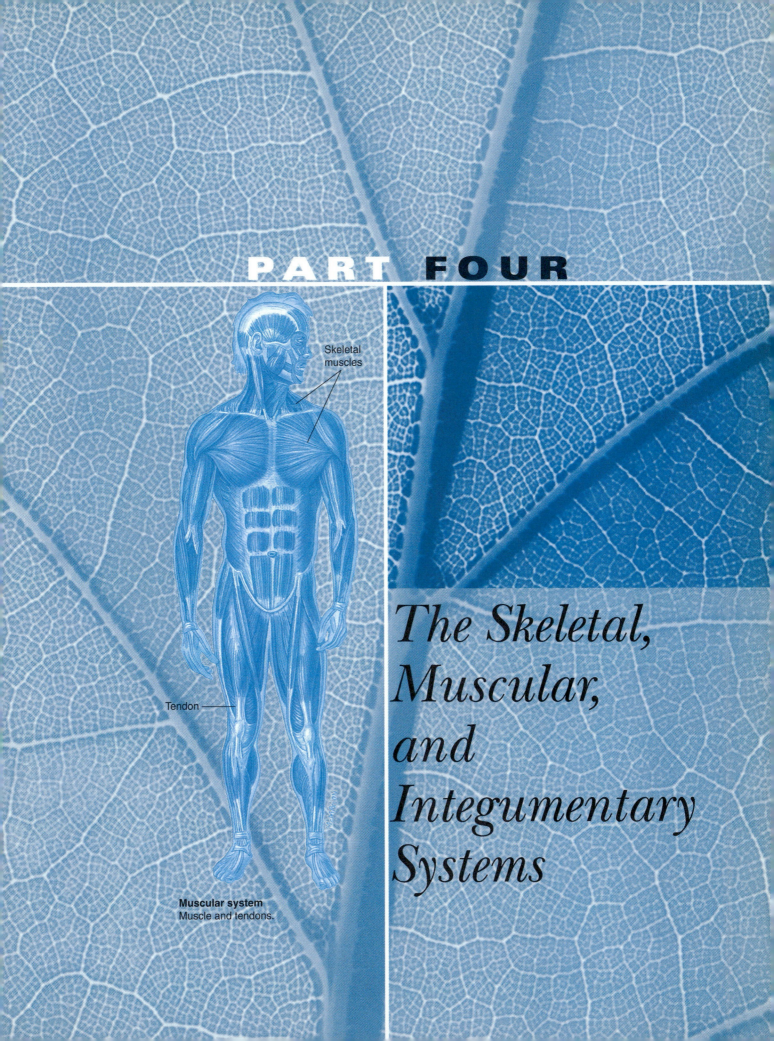

PART FOUR

Skeletal muscles

Tendon

Muscular system
Muscle and tendons.

The Skeletal, Muscular, and Integumentary Systems

Julie

GENDER	**SOCIOECONOMIC**
F	■ Middle class
AGE	**SPIRITUAL**
5	
SETTING	**PHARMACOLOGIC**
■ Hospital	■ Fentanyl (Sublimaze)
ETHNICITY	**PSYCHOSOCIAL**
■ Asian American	■ Family anxiety
CULTURAL CONSIDERATIONS	■ Grief
	LEGAL
PREEXISTING CONDITIONS	
■ Burns	**ETHICAL**
COEXISTING CONDITIONS	
	ALTERNATIVE THERAPY
SIGNIFICANT HISTORY	
	PRIORITIZATION
COMMUNICATION	■ Yes
	DELEGATION
DISABILITY	■ Yes

THE SKELETAL SYSTEM

Level of difficulty: Difficult

Overview: This case requires knowledge of burns and related care, the grief response, the client's background and personal situation as well as the mother–child attachment relationship.

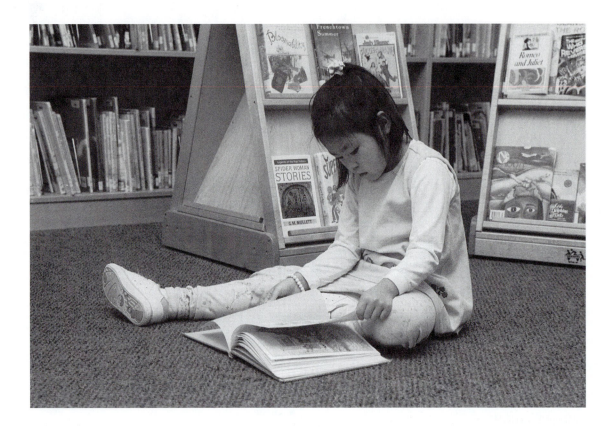

Client Profile

Julie is a 5-year-old girl who lives in North Carolina with her parents and two siblings, a 3-year-old brother and an 18-month-old sister. Her father works at a brokerage firm in Raleigh and her mother stays at home to care for the children. Julie has never had any health problems other than occasional episodes of the common cold.

Case Study

Julie and her parents were returning home from a family visit 4 weeks ago when they were involved in a motor vehicle accident resulting in an explosion that caused their car to become engulfed in flames. Julie's mother, who was sitting in the back seat with the children, perished in the fire while trying to save the children. Her father and two younger siblings escaped serious injury; however, Julie sustained third-degree burns over 80% of her body and was admitted to the Jaycee Burn Center. She was intubated and placed on mechanical ventilation. Currently she is no longer on mechanical ventilation and has a tracheostomy from which the nursing staff suctions thick green-yellow secretions every 2 to 3 hours. Julie is receiving total parenteral nutrition (TPN) and intralipids (IL) through a central venous access. Julie has severe wounds to her face, neck, left arm (necessitating the amputation of her left hand), left leg (necessitating a below-the-knee amputation), and back requiring extensive wound and graft care. She is premedicated with intravenous fentanyl prior to each dressing change, and this provides adequate pain management for these procedures.

Julie's father visits frequently. Julie is aware of the death of her mother and tends to be withdrawn and has had episodes of crying during which she could not be consoled.

Questions

1. Discuss the classifications and types of burns and how burns are measured to determine the percentage of body surface area involved.

2. Identify the negative and positive factors affecting Julie's prognosis and her chances of survival.

3. Why is Julie at high risk for developing an infection?

4. Discuss Julie's needs regarding her tracheostomy.

5. Discuss TPN, including general care and special nutritional needs of children with burn injuries.

6. What is the relationship between Julie's fluid and electrolyte balance and her burn status?

7. Discuss why fentanyl has been chosen for pain management for Julie's dressing changes.

8. Discuss how Julie's level of growth and development could affect her ability to cope with her mother's death.

9. What nursing interventions could help Julie cope with her hospitalization?

10. Discuss how you might feel in this situation if you were Julie's father.

Lauren

GENDER

F

AGE

Neonate

SETTING

■ Hospital/clinic

ETHNICITY

■ White American

CULTURAL CONSIDERATIONS

PREEXISTING CONDITIONS

COEXISTING CONDITIONS

SIGNIFICANT HISTORY

COMMUNICATION

DISABILITY

SOCIOECONOMIC

SPIRITUAL

PHARMACOLOGIC

PSYCHOSOCIAL

■ New parent anxiety

LEGAL

ETHICAL

ALTERNATIVE THERAPY

PRIORITIZATION

■ Yes

DELEGATION

■ Yes

THE SKELETAL SYSTEM

Level of difficulty: Easy

Overview: This case requires knowledge of congenital hip dysplagia, normal growth and development, as well as an understanding of the client's personal situation and mother–child attachment relationship.

Client Profile

Lauren is a neonate admitted into the newborn nursery after her breech vaginal delivery. She is the first child of a 25-year-old couple who have been anxiously awaiting Lauren's birth. Lauren's mother successfully breastfed her immediately after Lauren was born.

Case Study

On admission to the nursery, Lauren is weighed and measured. She weighs 4.5 kg (9 lb, 14 oz) and measures 55 cm (22 in.) in length. Her vital signs are within normal ranges; her skin color is pink and she is crying. The nurse notes no murmur when he listens to her heart and her bowel sounds are present. As the assessment continues, the nurse notes asymmetry of Lauren's thigh and gluteal folds and limited right hip abduction. Her right upper leg appears shorter than her left.

Questions

1. Discuss the significance of Lauren's clinical manifestations.

2. Discuss the potential causes Lauren's musculoskeletal manifestations.

3. What other assessment data would be helpful for the nurse to have to prepare Lauren's care plan?

4. Lauren is diagnosed with developmental dysplasia of the hip (DDH). Describe this condition, including the different types.

5. What is the incidence of DDH?

6. Lauren has subluxation DDH. What are the priorities of care for Lauren prior to discharge?

7. Lauren is referred to a pediatric orthopedist who recommends medical treatment for Lauren.

She is fitted for an orthopedic device. What is this device and how does it work?

8. What are the priorities of care for Lauren after she is fitted with the device?

9. Lauren's mother asks if she will still be able to breast feed Lauren after the harness is placed. What is the nurse's best response to this question?

10. Discuss the teaching necessary for Lauren's mother before she takes Lauren home with the device.

11. Discuss the impact of Lauren's condition on her growth and development.

Jason

GENDER	**SOCIOECONOMIC**
M	■ Middle class
AGE	**SPIRITUAL**
13	
SETTING	**PHARMACOLOGIC**
■ Emergency department	
ETHNICITY	**PSYCHOSOCIAL**
■ White American	■ Possible abuse
CULTURAL CONSIDERATIONS	**LEGAL**
	■ Mandatory reporting
PREEXISTING CONDITIONS	**ETHICAL**
	■ Child abuse
	■ Possible nurse bias
COEXISTING CONDITIONS	**ALTERNATIVE THERAPY**
SIGNIFICANT HISTORY	**PRIORITIZATION**
COMMUNICATION	**DELEGATION**
	■ Yes
DISABILITY	

THE SKELETAL SYSTEM

Level of difficulty: Moderate

Overview: This case requires knowledge of growth and development, as well as an understanding of the client's background, personal situation, parent–child attachment relationship, child abuse, and legal and ethical implications for nursing.

Client Profile

Jason is a 13-year-old adolescent who lives with his mother, father, 10-year-old sister, and 5-year-old brother in a middle-class rural neighborhood. Jason attends middle school and has been an average student, although he has demonstrated both attendance and behavior problems beginning 3 months ago. Teachers have suspected his difficulties stem from problems at home, but Jason denies this. They have noted that Jason appears in pain when sitting in class, especially on Mondays, that he is regularly absent, and that most of his absences occur on Mondays. He has been suspended twice this school year for being involved in altercations with other students on school property. Jason's mother attends all parent conferences and when these observations were communicated to her, she responded that Jason and his father were "not getting along very well." When teachers suggested that it would be beneficial to speak to both his mother and father, Mrs. King responded that her husband was "frequently gone in the afternoons and evenings and that any communications from the school should be made directly with her."

Case Study

Mrs. King brings Jason to the emergency room at 0100 after "he fell down the stairs at home." His breathing suggests a patent airway, however, he is bleeding from both nares. When the nurse attempts to apply pressure to Jason's nose to stop the bleeding, Jason grimaces and rates his pain level at 10/10, complaining of pain in his right arm as well as the bridge of his nose. During his triage assessment, the nurse notes the following:

Vital signs:

Temperature: 37° C (98.6° F)

Pulse: 98 beats/minute

Respirations: 30 breaths/minute

Blood pressure: 128/88

Breath sounds clear to auscultation

Heart sounds regular with no audible dysrhythmias or murmurs

Areas of ecchymosis on upper arms bilaterally

Displacement of the bridge of the nose to the right and bleeding from the nares

Guarding of his right forearm

Neurological assessment reveals no apparent deficits.

Skin assessment revealed multiple horizontal lacerations across Jason's back from the thoracic area extending down to and including his buttocks bilaterally. In addition, 2.5-cm (1-in.) wide horizontal scars were also noted in this area. Jason states that he had awakened at "about midnight" and fell when he was walking to the bathroom in his home. Although both Jason and his mother are cooperative during the history-taking, the nurse notes that neither makes eye contact with the nurse, but rather keep looking at each other during the interview. As Jason is in no acute distress, the nurse leaves the triage room to report his findings to the health care provider on call in the emergency room.

Questions

1. Discuss your impressions about the above situation.

2. What data obtained by the nurse are most pertinent regarding the client's present condition?

3. What additional data would be helpful in determining the extent of Jason's injuries?

4. Jason is diagnosed with a complete closed fracture of the right ulna and nasal septum, and multiple skin lacerations. Identify four priority goals of care for Jason during triage.

5. Discuss interventions to achieve the identified priority goals.

6. What referrals should be implemented in this situation and why are they appropriate?

7. Jason's mother begins to cry and states that she is afraid her husband "is going to be mad because I brought Jason to the hospital and our insurance doesn't cover emergency room fees." How should you respond to her and the concerns she has voiced?

8. What client and family teaching should be completed prior to Jason's discharge from the emergency department to home?

9. Discuss your own biases about this situation.

10. What are the benefits and risks of delaying judgment about the father's potential involvement in Jason's condition until all the data and facts are available?

Kimberli

GENDER

F

AGE

11

SETTING

- Health care provider's office/hospital

ETHNICITY

- White American

CULTURAL CONSIDERATIONS

PREEXISTING CONDITIONS

COEXISTING CONDITIONS

SIGNIFICANT HISTORY

COMMUNICATION

DISABILITY

SOCIOECONOMIC

SPIRITUAL

PHARMACOLOGIC

- Pain management

PSYCHOSOCIAL

- Client anxiety
- Disturbed body image

LEGAL

ETHICAL

ALTERNATIVE THERAPY

PRIORITIZATION

- Yes

DELEGATION

MODERATE

THE SKELETAL SYSTEM

Level of difficulty: Moderate

Overview: This case requires knowledge of scoliosis, medical–surgical treatment, growth and development, as well as an understanding of the client's background, personal situation, and family–child attachment relationship.

Client Profile

Kimberli is an 11-year-old school-age child who lives with her parents and 13-year-old brother in a suburban community. She attends school and performs well. During her last physical examination for school, her pediatrician expressed concern about Kimberli's posture, which had a slight right lateral curve. X-ray studies were done at this time. The health care provider instructed Kimberli and Kimberli's parents to encourage proper posture and inform him if they notice any worsening of her condition. The radiological report indicated that Kimberli's curvature was <20%.

Case Study

During a subsequent visit, Kimberli's curvature appears worse and a spinal X-ray film is prescribed. The x-ray indicates the presence of a >30% lateral curvature of the spinal column at the level of T4–T11. Scoliometric measurements and magnetic resonance imaging (MRI) confirms that Kimberli has scoliosis of unknown etiology. Her diagnosis and treatment plan is explained to Kimberli and her parents.

Questions

1. Describe scoliosis, including the different types.

2. Discuss the incidence and etiology of idiopathic scoliosis.

3. How might her diagnosis impact on Kimberli's growth and development?

4. Describe the medical treatment for idiopathic scoliosis.

5. Discuss the teaching required for Kimberli and her parents in relation to her medical treatment.

6. After Kimberli's scoliosis does not respond to conservative treatment, she is scheduled for a posterior spinal fusion. What are the priorities of care for Kimberli prior to surgery?

7. What is a Harrington rod and how is it used during spinal fusion surgery?

8. Following her surgery, what are the postoperative priorities of care for Kimberli?

9. Pulse oximetry reveals that Kimberli's oxygen saturation is 89%. She is receiving 2 L of oxygen per nasal cannula. Discuss the appropriate actions the nurse should take.

10. Discuss the importance of pain management for Kimberli and what agent(s) you anticipate will be prescribed to control her surgical pain.

11. Discuss the nursing interventions necessary to prevent complications of Kimberli's surgery.

12. Kimberli has been working with a physical therapist for 3 days and on her 5th postoperative day, you are preparing to get Kimberli out of bed and help her to the chair. What nursing interventions are necessary before getting Kimberli out of bed?

13. Kimberli has not had a bowel movement since her surgery and complains of abdominal fullness. Discuss your impressions of Kimberli's situation including factors that may have precipitated her present condition and the nursing interventions that are appropriate at this time.

GENDER

M

AGE

14

SETTING

- Hospital

ETHNICITY

- Russian

CULTURAL CONSIDERATIONS

- Recent Russian immigrant

PREEXISTING CONDITIONS

- Osteogenic sarcoma
- Implanted CVAD

COEXISTING CONDITIONS

SIGNIFICANT HISTORY

- Immigrant

COMMUNICATION

- Russian-speaking

DISABILITY

SOCIOECONOMIC

- Middle class

SPIRITUAL

PHARMACOLOGIC

- Methotrexate (Trexall)
- Prednisone (Deltasone)
- Doxorubicin (Rubex)

PSYCHOSOCIAL

- Impaired verbal communication
- Anxiety

LEGAL

ETHICAL

ALTERNATIVE THERAPY

PRIORITIZATION

- Yes

DELEGATION

- Graduate nurse and preceptor

THE SKELETAL SYSTEM

Level of difficulty: Difficult

Overview: This case requires knowledge of osteogenic sarcoma, growth and development, an understanding of the client's background, personal situation, and family relationship, and how to work with non-English-speaking clients.

DIFFICULT

Client Profile

Ilya is a 14-year-old Russian boy who recently came to the United States to receive treatment for osteogenic sarcoma (OS) of his right femur. He was diagnosed 2 months ago in his home country, where he had undergone chemotherapy. His father is a contractor who has worked in the United States for 2 years with plans to have his family join him soon. After his son was diagnosed with OS, he brought Ilya and the boy's mother to the United States for further treatment in a research facility that he has been unable to receive in his home country. Ilya is admitted to the hospital for a limb-sparing surgical procedure. He has an implanted central venous access device (CVAD) through which he received chemotherapy during to his earlier hospital admission in his home country. The health care provider prescribes continuation of his chemotherapy regimen. Ilya and his mother do not speak English; however, his father, who is fluent in English as well as Russian, is present on admission and provides the nurse with Ilya's medical and social history and translates information for his wife and son. Ilya appears to be a happy and otherwise healthy adolescent whose psychosocial and physical development is appropriate for his age.

Case Study

Ilya is continuing his chemotherapy regime of methotrexate, prednisone, and doxorubicin prior to surgery which is scheduled 3 days from now. His current diagnostic findings are:

Hematology:

Hemoglobin: 10.6 g/dL

Hematocrit: 30%

White blood cell count: 8,900 cells/mm^3 with a differential of:

Neutrophils: 21%

Lymphocytes: 65%

Eosinophils: 4%

Bands: 1%

Monocytes: 7%

Platelets: 90,000 cells/mm^3

Chemistry:

Potassium: 3.2 mEq/L

Sodium: 130 mEq/L

Glucose: 260 mg/dL

Calcium: 8.1 mg/dL

Uric acid: 6.3 mg/dL

In making assignments for the pediatric unit where Ilya is a client, the charge nurse assigns him to a new graduate nurse, Sally, who is orienting to the unit and Sally's preceptor, John, who has worked on this pediatric oncology unit for 2 years. Sally is excited about working with Ilya and hopes to help him learn some English while she improves her Russian, learned while she was an exchange student in high school.

Questions

1. Discuss your impressions of Ilya's laboratory findings.

2. Identify the nursing concerns related to these findings.

3. Ilya's father is unable to visit on a regular basis because of his job. Identify nursing concerns related to the language barrier in this situation when the client's father is not present.

4. Why do you think the charge nurse should or should not assign Ilya to the new graduate and her preceptor? Discuss both the benefits and disadvantages.

5. Discuss the incidence and prognosis of osteogenic sarcoma.

6. What are the surgical standards of care for a child with this condition?

7. Discuss the appropriate priority nursing interventions for Ilya to prevent the complications associated with his chemotherapy regimen.

8. What are Ilya's risk factors for developing an infection?

9. How will the nurse know if Ilya develops an infection?

10. Five days following his limb-sparing surgery, Ilya's White blood cell count is 6,000 cells/mm,^{3} his neutrophil count is 49%, and, following transfusion of 2 units of platelets, his platelet count is 120,000. Following the nurse's assessment, Ilya communicates with Sally in broken English that he misses his friends in Russia and would like to make some new friends here. Discuss your impressions of Ilya's request based on his level of growth and development.

11. John notes that Ilya's mother remains constantly at his bedside and is weepy at times when Ilya is in the adolescent activity room. John has a friend who studied Russian as his second language while he was working on a computer account in Russia. He asks the friend, Brett, to come to the hospital and visit with Ilya's mother. What do you think is John's rationale for this?

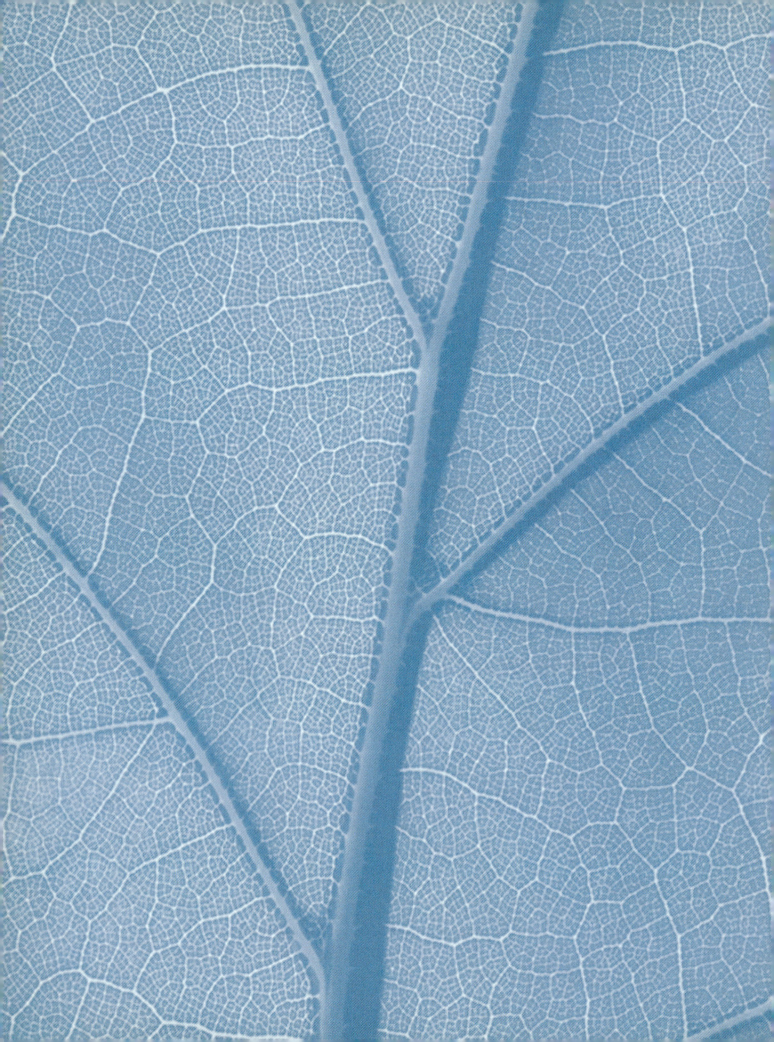

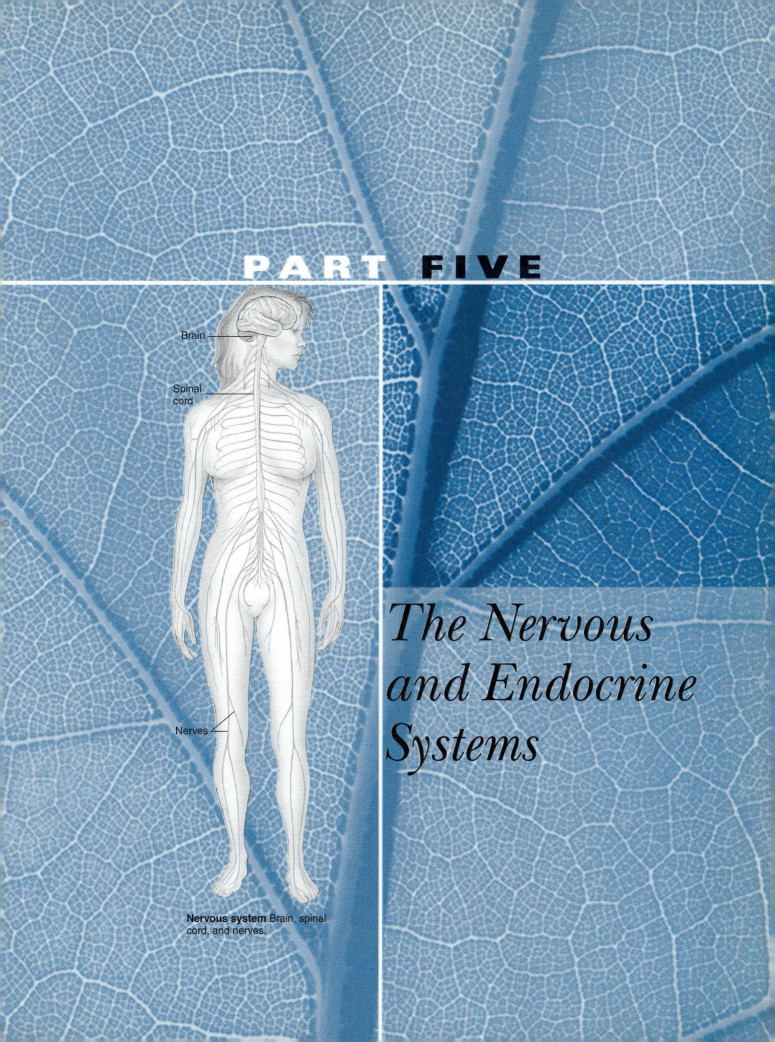

PART FIVE

Brain

Spinal
cord

Nerves

Nervous system Brain, spinal
cord, and nerves.

The Nervous
and Endocrine
Systems

Andrea

GENDER	**SOCIOECONOMIC**
F	■ Middle class
AGE	**SPIRITUAL**
7	
SETTING	**PHARMACOLOGIC**
■ Health care provider's office	■ Levothyroxine sodium (Synthoid)
ETHNICITY	**PSYCHOSOCIAL**
■ Spanish American	
CULTURAL CONSIDERATIONS	**LEGAL**
PREEXISTING CONDITIONS	**ETHICAL**
■ Congenital hypothyroidism	
COEXISTING CONDITIONS	**ALTERNATIVE THERAPY**
SIGNIFICANT HISTORY	**PRIORITIZATION**
	■ Yes
COMMUNICATION	**DELEGATION**
	■ Yes
DISABILITY	

THE ENDOCRINE SYSTEM

Level of difficulty: Easy

Overview: This case requires knowledge of thyroid dysfunction, growth and development, as well as an understanding of the client's background, personal situation, and mother–child attachment relationship.

Client Profile

Andrea was 3.6 kg (8 lb) and was 50 cm (20 in.) long when she was born. At 2 months of age, she was diagnosed with congenital hypothyroidism. She is now 7 years old and lives with her mother and two siblings. Since her diagnosis she has been treated with levothyroxine. She sees her pediatrician every 6 months for follow-up and at her visit 6 weeks ago her dosage was increased to 125 mcg once every day. She enjoys school and earns a "B" average. For the past month Andrea has experienced difficulty in school and her mother notices that Andrea is irritable and has trouble keeping her attention focussed on tasks that normally would not cause any difficulty. She has problems sleeping and for the past week has experienced daily bouts of diarrhea. Her mother makes an appointment with Andrea's pediatrician.

Case Study

Andrea is brought to the pediatrician's office by her mother. The office nurse greets Andrea and her mother and notes that Andrea is fidgety and has difficulty focusing on the nurse's questions. Andrea's vital signs are: Temperature, 37.8° C (100° F); pulse, 120 beats/minute; respirations, 28 breaths/minute; and blood pressure, 116/76. She weighs 55 lb and is 112.5 cm (45 in.) tall. Her mother explains that Andrea has had diarrhea for the past week. During the nursing history, Andrea's mother tells the nurse about the other changes that she has noted in her daughter over the past month.

Questions

1. What is congenital hypothyroidism?

2. Discuss the clinical manifestations of congenital hypothyroidism.

3. What is the incidence of congenital hypothyroidism and why is it important to diagnose this condition as soon as possible after birth?

4. Discuss the significance of Andrea's clinical manifestations and their possible causes.

5. Discuss the significance of Andrea's vital signs.

6. What other assessment data would be helpful for the nurse to have to prepare Andrea's care plan?

7. What are the priorities of care for Andrea during this office visit?

8. The safe dosage range of levothyroxine is 4–5 mcg/kg per day. Is Andrea's currently prescribed dosage safe for her?

9. Discuss your impressions of why Andrea's mother did not bring Andrea's other clinical manifestations to the pediatrician's attention earlier.

10. How do you anticipate the pediatrician will treat Andrea's current condition?

11. Discuss the teaching priorities for Andrea and her mother prior to discharge from the office today.

Brent

GENDER

M

AGE

9

SETTING

- School/hospital

ETHNICITY

- White American

CULTURAL CONSIDERATIONS

PREEXISTING CONDITIONS

- Motor vehicle accident (MVA) or motor vehicle crash (MVC)/closed head injury (CHI)

COEXISTING CONDITIONS

SIGNIFICANT HISTORY

COMMUNICATION

DISABILITY

- Seizures

SOCIOECONOMIC

- Middle class

SPIRITUAL

PHARMACOLOGIC

- Phenytoin sodium (Dilatin)

PSYCHOSOCIAL

- Client anxiety
- Parent anxiety

LEGAL

ETHICAL

ALTERNATIVE THERAPY

PRIORITIZATION

DELEGATION

THE ENDOCRINE SYSTEM

Level of difficulty: Moderate

Overview: This case requires knowledge of seizures, growth and development, as well as an understanding of the client's background, personal situation, and parent–child relationship.

Client Profile

Brent is a 9-year-old schoolage child who lives with his parents and two siblings. He attends middle school and achieves average performance. Last year Brent and his family were involved in a motor vehicle accident in which Brent experienced a closed head injury. He was hospitalized for 3 months and through therapy has regained his mobility, cognitive functioning, and most of his memory. During his recovery he experienced several seizures and was prescribed phenytoin sodium 50 mg PO t.i.d. When he returned to school, his parents informed the school nurse of Brent's condition. Brent takes one dose of medication before school, one at lunchtime, and the last dose in the evening at home. This regimen has controlled his seizure activity.

Case Study

This afternoon at school, Brent experiences a seizure involving loss of consciousness, violent spasms, and stiffening with the upper extremities flexed and the lower extremities extended. His classroom teacher moved all the desks away from where Brent was having his seizure, placed a pillow under his head, and sent one of the other students in her class to bring the school nurse to the classroom. By the time the nurse arrived at the classroom about 2 minutes later, Brent's seizure was over and he was lying quietly on the floor. The nurse was able to arouse him and sent the teacher to the office to call 911. His parents were called, and he was transferred to the local acute care facility.

Questions

1. What are seizures?

2. Discuss the different types of seizures that affect children.

3. How common are seizures in children and what causes them?

4. Discuss the significance of the characteristics of Brent's seizure.

5. Discuss the possible relationship between Brent's closed head injury and the development of seizures.

6. What assessment data would be helpful for the nurse to have to prepare Brent's care plan on admission?

7. What are the priorities of care for Brent on admission?

8. What is phenytoin sodium and why is Brent prescribed this medication?

9. Brent's phenytoin sodium level is 4 mcg/mL. Discuss this level and what actions the nurse should take as a result of this information.

10. Brent weighs 30 kg (66 lb) on admission. Following diagnostic testing, his health care provider increases Brent's dosage of phenytoin sodium to 75 mg PO t.i.d. Discuss the rationale for this change and whether this dose is within the safe dosage range.

11. What impact might Brent's seizure condition have on his growth and development?

12. Discuss the teaching priorities for Brent and his parents as he prepares for discharge from the hospital.

Jessica

GENDER

F

AGE

13

SETTING

- Hospital

ETHNICITY

- White American

CULTURAL CONSIDERATIONS

PREEXISTING CONDITIONS

- Type I diabetes

COEXISTING CONDITIONS

SIGNIFICANT HISTORY

COMMUNICATION

DISABILITY

SOCIOECONOMIC

- Middle class

SPIRITUAL

PHARMACOLOGIC

- NPH Humulin insulin
- 5% Dextrose

PSYCHOSOCIAL

LEGAL

ETHICAL

ALTERNATIVE THERAPY

PRIORITIZATION

- Yes

DELEGATION

- Yes

THE ENDOCRINE SYSTEM

Level of difficulty: Moderate

Overview: This case requires knowledge of diabetes mellitus, nutritional needs of adolescence, as well as an understanding of the client's background, personal situation, and family relationship.

Client Profile

Jessica is a 13-year-old high school student who lives with her parents and younger brother Jonathan (11 years old) in a middle-class neighborhood. Both Mr. and Mrs. Morris work in the community where they live. Jessica has had diabetes mellitus type 1 insulin dependent diabetes mellitus (IDDM) since the age of 7, which has been well controlled with morning and evening injections of NPH Humulin insulin, diet, and exercise. Jessica has been staying up later in the evenings studying for her end-of-year (EOY) exams, and is also the pitcher on her school's softball team, which is playing in the semifinals. Her heavy schedule has contributed to changes in her eating and sleeping habits.

Case Study

Jessica developed a cough, nasal congestion, and a low-grade temperature 3 days ago, but told her parents she felt well enough to go to school and didn't want to miss any of her classes or softball practice. Today Jessica felt worse, so her mother called Jessica's pediatrician, Dr. Sheila Jones, who told Mrs. Morris to bring Jessica into her office. Dr. Jones recommended that Mrs. Morris take Jessica to the emergency department of the hospital, at which point she noted that Jessica's pulse and respirations were elevated, her breath had a fruity odor, and her capillary blood sugar level was elevated. At the emergency department, Jessica's diagnostic test findings are as follows:

Chemistry profile: glucose, 480 mg/dL; sodium, 130 mEq/L; chloride, 79 mEq/L; and potassium, 3.3 mEq/L

Arterial blood gases: pH, 7. 19; $Paco_2$, 25 mm Hg; HCO_3, 10 mEq/L; Pao_2, 92 mm Hg; oxygen saturation, 97%

Questions

1. Discuss your impressions about the above situation.

2. How do you explain the abnormal values of Jessica's arterial blood gases?

3. What data indicate that Jessica's lungs are attempting to compensate for her present condition?

4. What factors place Jessica at risk for diabetic ketoacidosis (DKA)?

5. What other data would be helpful to determine whether she has developed other complications of either her DKA or her flu-like symptoms?

6. What medical management should you be prepared to initiate for Jessica?

7. After Jessica has received 2 L of intravenous fluids and her blood glucose level decreases 240 mg/dL, the health care provider prescribes adding 5% dextrose to her intravenous solution. Should you question this prescription? Why or why not?

8. What other medical management interventions would you expect to be prescribed to facilitate Jessica's recovery?

9. Discuss the potential complications for Jessica if she is not compliant with her medical regimen when she goes home.

10. In collaboration with the health care provider, what referrals might you obtain prior to Jessica's discharge?

11. What are the teaching priorities for Jessica and her parents prior to discharge?

Melanie

GENDER

F

AGE

16

SETTING

- Psychiatric unit

ETHNICITY

- White American

CULTURAL CONSIDERATIONS

PREEXISTING CONDITIONS

COEXISTING CONDITIONS

SIGNIFICANT HISTORY

- Interrupted relationships

COMMUNICATION

DISABILITY

SOCIOECONOMIC

SPIRITUAL

PHARMACOLOGIC

PSYCHOSOCIAL

- Recent parent separation
- Recent break-up with boyfriend

LEGAL

- Physical restraints

ETHICAL

ALTERNATIVE THERAPY

PRIORITIZATION

- Yes

DELEGATION

THE NERVOUS SYSTEM

Level of difficulty: Moderate

Overview: This case requires knowledge of anger issues, growth and development, as well as an understanding of the client's background, personal situation, and family–child relationship.

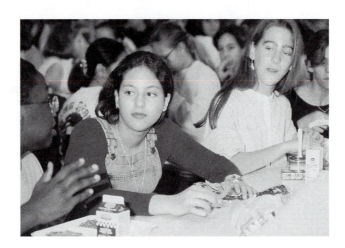

Client Profile

Melanie is a 16-year-old who lived with her parents and two siblings in a suburban neighborhood until her parents separated 6 months ago. At that time her school performance began to decline and she was truant from school, frequently not returning home until after dark. When she arrived home, she was verbally abusive to her mother when asked where she had been. Three days ago, her relationship with her boyfriend of 1 year ended when he told her she had "changed" and he didn't know how to "relate to her anymore." That evening, Melanie became very disruptive at home, breaking lamps and mirrors and turning over furniture. When her mother attempted to talk to Melanie, her daughter threatened her. Melanie was admitted to the children's psychiatric unit of the local inpatient mental health facility.

Case Study

Since her admission, Melanie has refused to attend any group sessions or talk to staff, and spends most of her time in her room. At change of shifts today, the staff heard a loud noise after which registered nurse and two psychiatric technologists (psych tech) rushed to Melanie's room. There they observed Melanie screaming incoherently and throwing chairs against the wall; clothes were littered across the floor.

Questions

1. Discuss your impression of the situation with Melanie.

2. What impact might Melanie's level of growth and development have on her response to life stressors?

3. What are the priorities of care for Melanie at this time?

4. What other assessment data would be helpful for the nurse to have to prepare Melanie's care plan?

5. What factors should the nurse consider prior to approaching Melanie?

6. When Melanie attempts the throw a chair at staff, the nurse supervisor determines that Melanie needs physical restraint. Discuss the supervisor's decision.

7. What precautions must be taken when physically restraining a client?

8. Do you think that Melanie's behavior at home warranted hospitalization?

9. Do you think her present behavior warrants continued hospitalization?

10. Discuss the advantages of waiting until all the data are available before making decisions about Melanie's course of treatment.

11. Melanie's mother calls the unit every day to check on her daughter but is not sure whether she should visit Melanie because, as she says, "I'm afraid I'll upset her. I think she feels that this whole situation is my fault. I love my daughter and I just want her to get well." How would you respond to Melanie's mother?

Andrew

GENDER

M

AGE

10

SETTING

- Hospital

ETHNICITY

- White American

CULTURAL CONSIDERATIONS

PREEXISTING CONDITIONS

- Motor vehicle accident (MVA)

COEXISTING CONDITIONS

SIGNIFICANT HISTORY

COMMUNICATION

DISABILITY

SOCIOECONOMIC

SPIRITUAL

PHARMACOLOGIC

- Ranitidine (Zantac)
- Metoclopramide (Maxolan)
- Phenytoin (Dilantin)

PSYCHOSOCIAL

- Parental anxiety

LEGAL

ETHICAL

ALTERNATIVE THERAPY

PRIORITIZATION

- Yes

DELEGATION

- Yes

DIFFICULT

THE NERVOUS SYSTEM

Level of difficulty: Difficult

Overview: This case requires knowledge of head trauma, increased intracranial pressure, growth and development and nutrition, as well as an understanding of the client's background, personal situation, and parent–child relationship.

Client Profile

Andrew is a 10-year-old fifth grader who lives with his parents in the suburb of a large city. He is active in school and enjoys playing with his neighborhood friends. His father (Randy) works in the city and his mother (Joyce) works part-time as a computer programmer from her home office. She takes Andrew to and from school each day and is active in all of his school and extracurricular activities. Andrew is an A–B student who enjoys his school subjects and wants to study to become a doctor one day. The family lives approximately 5 miles from his school. Mr. Burger also is very involved in his son's activities.

Case Study

After picking up Andrew at school 3 weeks ago, Mrs. Burger was involved in a serious motor vehicle accident while driving home. Both she and Andrew had their seat belt restraints fastened. The accident occurred when a van did not stop for a stoplight and struck their car in the side where Andrew was riding. Mrs. Burger sustained lacerations from broken window glass, but Andrew received a closed head injury from the impact. Mrs. Burger was treated in the emergency department of the city hospital and released; however, Andrew was admitted to the pediatric intensive care unit. He was nonresponsive at the scene of the accident, and on admission his Glasgow Coma Scale score was 3 out of 15. He was transferred to the pediatric nursing unit last week. A CD player at his bedside plays music. He focuses and tracks as his parents talk to him, and they perform most of his care, including range-of-motion exercises twice a day. He is receiving oxygen via a tracheostomy collar. He coughs up most of his respiratory secretions, but still requires suctioning every 3–4 hours. He receives enteral nutrition through his gastrostomy tube. This is the first day you have been assigned to Andrew, and during your assessment you find the client awake and able to respond by nodding and shaking his head for "yes" and "no" when questioned. He moves his extremities spontaneously and on command; however, you note bilateral weakness. His Glasgow Coma Scale score currently is 4–1–5, his vital signs are within normal limits for his age, he weighs 77 lb, and is 1.5 m (5 ft) tall. His lungs are clear bilaterally and his bowel sounds are present on all four quadrants. He remains incontinent of urine and stool. You overhear Andrew's mother tell him she is "so sorry" about the accident and she begins to cry softly.

Questions

1. Discuss the priorities of care for Andrew on his admission to the pediatric critical care unit.

2. What were the priority nursing interventions for Andrew on his admission to the PICU?

3. What is the meaning and significance of Andrew's Glasgow Coma Scale score on admission?

4. Discuss the differences between the Glasgow Coma Scale used for infants and children and the Glasgow Coma Scale used for adults and which one is the most appropriate one to use when assessing Andrew.

5. Why do you think Andrew has a tracheostomy?

6. Discuss your impressions as to why Andrew receives enteral feedings.

7. Why is the radio placed at Andrew's bedside?

8. Discuss Andrew's current Glasgow Coma Scale score.

9. What are your nursing priorities for Andrew following your assessment?

10. Why is it important that Andrew receive range-of-motion exercises?

11. What risk factors predispose Andrew to infection?

12. Andrew receives all of his medications via his G-tube and is prescribed ranitidine 70 mg per G-tube b.i.d., metoclopramide 3.5 mg q.i.d., and phenytoin 70 mg b.i.d. Discuss Andrew's medications related to why he is receiving each medication, the safety of the dosages prescribed, and any special precautions needed related to route of administration.

13. What is your priority concern about Andrew's urinary and bowel incontinence?

14. How would you explain Mrs. Burger's comments to Andrew and what might your therapeutic interventions consist of?

15. How can you intervene to help meet Andrew's growth and development needs?

16. What other health care professionals would be beneficial in Andrew's care?

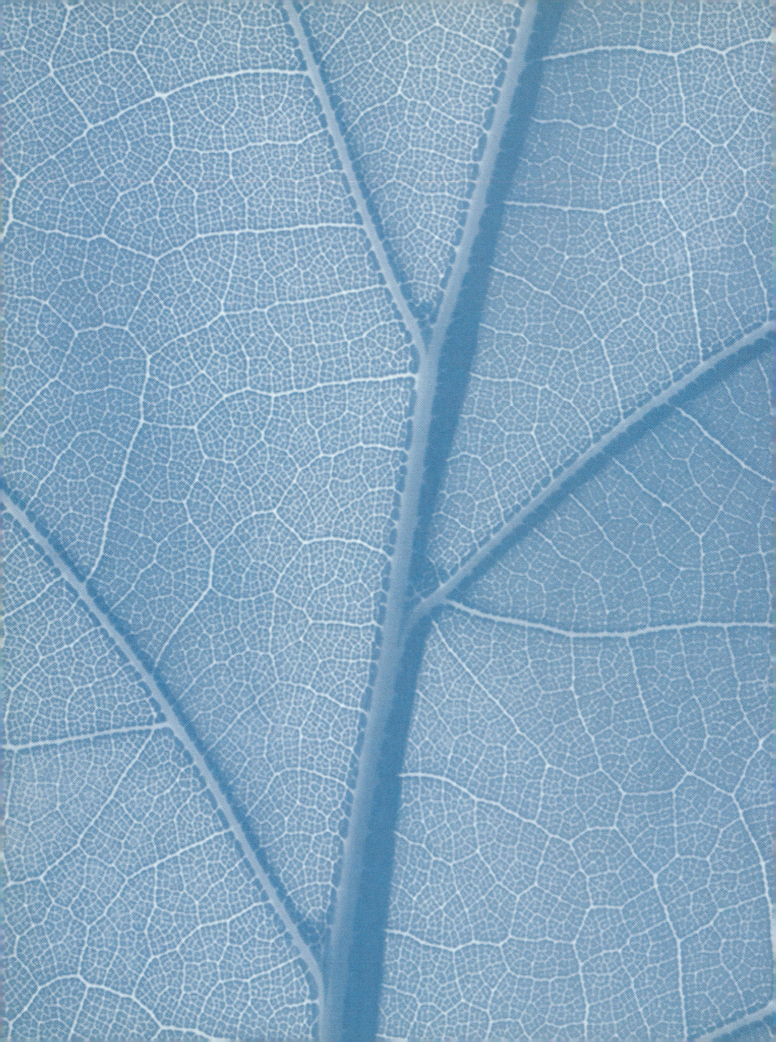

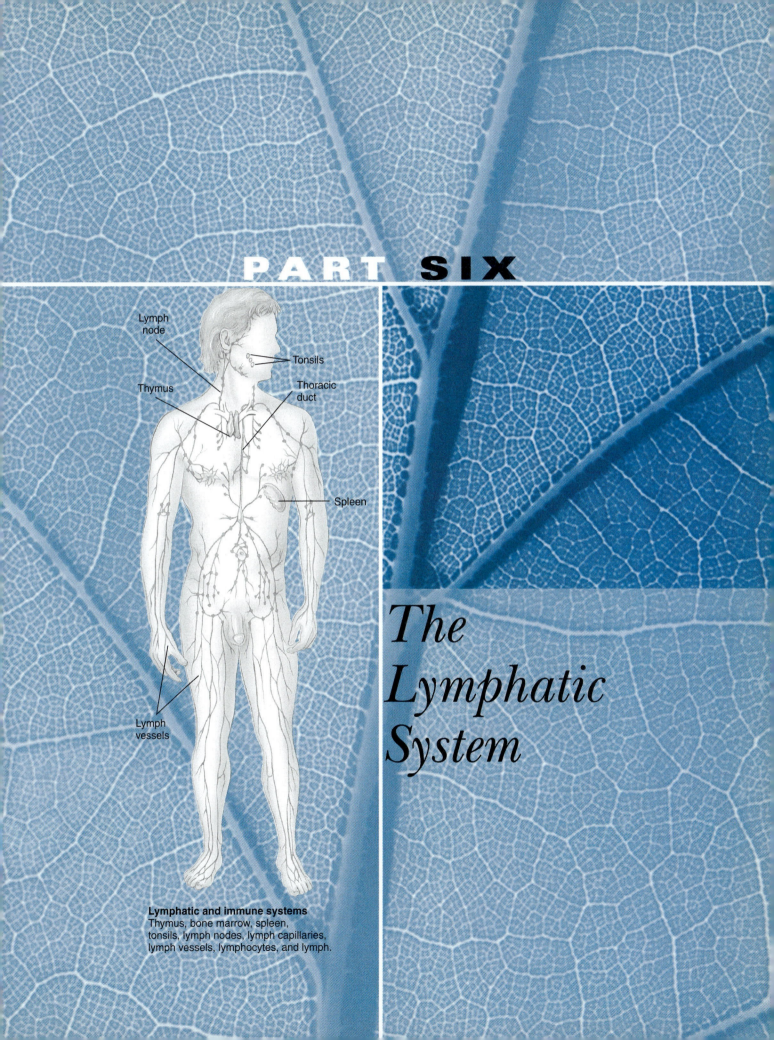

PART SIX

Lymph
node

Tonsils

Thymus

Thoracic
duct

Spleen

Lymph
vessels

Lymphatic and immune systems
Thymus, bone marrow, spleen,
tonsils, lymph nodes, lymph capillaries,
lymph vessels, lymphocytes, and lymph.

The
Lymphatic
System

David

GENDER

M

AGE

20

SETTING

■ Hospital/home

ETHNICITY

■ White American

CULTURAL CONSIDERATIONS

PREEXISTING CONDITIONS

COEXISTING CONDITIONS

■ Hodgkin's disease

SIGNIFICANT HISTORY

■ Lives with wife

COMMUNICATION

DISABILITY

SOCIOECONOMIC

SPIRITUAL

■ Jehovah Witness

PHARMACOLOGIC

■ Cyclophosphamide (Cytoxan)

PSYCHOSOCIAL

■ Death and dying

LEGAL

■ Client's right to die
■ Do not resuscitate order

ETHICAL

■ Client's right to die
■ Possible nurse bias

ALTERNATIVE THERAPY

PRIORITIZATION

■ Yes

DELEGATION

■ Yes

THE LYMPHATIC SYSTEM

Level of difficulty: Easy

Overview: This case requires knowledge of Hodgkin's disease, chemotherapy, spiritual integrity, growth and development, as well as an understanding of the client's background, personal situation, and marital relationship.

Client Profile

David is a 20-year-old who lives with his wife in a metropolitan area. He received an associate degree in business from a community college and works with his father in the family hardware business. David and his wife are Jehovah Witnesses. Two years ago David was diagnosed with Hodgkin's disease and was treated with chemotherapy. He achieved remission for 18 months, at which time his disease relapsed. For the past 3 months, he has been receiving chemotherapy but has not been able to achieve remission. He has been hospitalized three times for chemotherapy and once for adverse effects of his chemotherapy regimen. Today David is experiencing gross bleeding when he urinates. When he sees his oncologist, the physician admits David to the pediatric oncology unit at the medical center where he has been undergoing treatment for his Hodgkin's disease.

Case Study

David and his wife arrive on the unit for placement of a three-way catheter, continuous bladder irrigation with sterile normal saline, continuous monitoring of oxygen saturation via pulse oximetry, administration of oxygen to maintain saturations >94%, intravenous fluids of lactated Ringer's solution to infuse at 200 mL/hour. His admitting vital signs are: temperature, 36° C (96.8° F); pulse, 110 beats/minute; respirations, 30 breaths/minute; and blood pressure, 90/60. His pulse oximetry

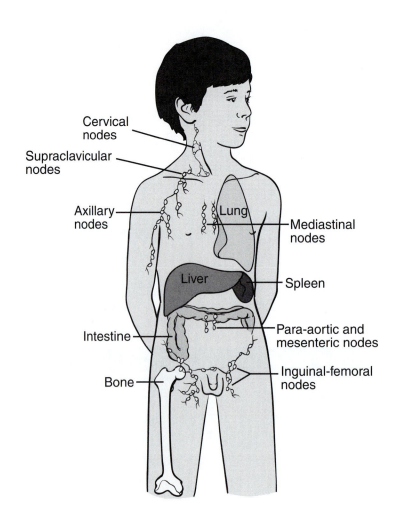

Lymph nodes affected by Hodgkin's disease

reading is 86%. He complains of weakness, dizziness, shortness of breath, and anxiety. His skin is cool and clammy. His admitting laboratory values are:

Complete blood count:

Hemoglobin: 9 g/dL

Hematocrit: 25%

Platelets: 80,000 cells/mm^3

White blood cell count: 4,000 cells/mm^3

His admitting history reveals that his chemotherapy regimen to treat his Hodgkin disease is the alkylating agent cyclophosphamide. His urine is bright red with occasional clots present. His wife is visibly anxious and states, "I am so afraid for David even though we have talked about his condition and that he might die as a result of it."

Questions

1. Discuss your impressions of David's clinical manifestations.

2. What is the significance of David's laboratory findings?

3. Discuss the relationship, if any, between David's present condition and his chemotherapy treatment.

4. What other assessment data would be helpful for the nurse to have to prepare David's care plan?

5. Discuss the rationales for what the oncologist has prescribed for David.

6. What are the priorities of care for David on admission?

7. How would you respond to David's wife and her concern?

8. What impact might David and his wife's spiritual beliefs have on his medical treatment plan?

9. The oncologist informs David and his wife that David needs a transfusion of packed red blood cells and explains why this treatment is necessary. They both refuse this treatment. Discuss your feelings and biases about their decision.

10. Discuss the legality of the decision made by David and his wife.

11. David's condition deteriorates as the continuous bladder irrigation is unable to stop the bleeding from his urinary bladder. He and his wife communicate to the oncologist that they don't want him resuscitated if he experiences cardiopulmonary arrest. The oncologist respects their request and initiates "Do Not Resuscitate" and "Discharge to Home" orders. Discuss your feelings about this decision.

12. What referrals might be helpful for David and his wife before he is discharged?

13. Later in the day, David is resting with his eyes closed when the nurse enters the room to do her discharge assessment. His wife says angrily, "Can't you people just leave us alone?" Discuss your impression of her comment and how you would respond to her.

14. Two weeks after David is discharged, he dies at home with his wife and parents at his bedside. His wife sends a card to the nursing unit to thank them for the "wonderful" care David received and that he had "died peacefully and with dignity." You notice that one of your nursing peers begins to weep. Discuss your feelings about the nurse's response and how you might interact with her.

GENDER

M

AGE

11

SETTING

- Hospital

ETHNICITY

- Black American

CULTURAL CONSIDERATIONS

PREEXISTING CONDITIONS

- Acute myelocytic leukemia

COEXISTING CONDITIONS

SIGNIFICANT HISTORY

COMMUNICATION

DISABILITY

SOCIOECONOMIC

SPIRITUAL

PHARMACOLOGIC

- Chemotherapy

PSYCHOSOCIAL

- Client anxiety
- Parent anxiety

LEGAL

- Informed consent

ETHICAL

- Assent

ALTERNATIVE THERAPY

PRIORITIZATION

- Yes

DELEGATION

- Yes

THE LYMPHATIC SYSTEM

Level of difficulty: Moderate

Overview: This case requires knowledge of leukemia, bone marrow transplantation, growth and development, as well as client's background and personal situation including family relationship.

Client Profile   **Jerome** is an 11-year-old middle-school child who lives at home with his 13-year-old brother Jason and their parents. Mr. and Mrs. Jones work full time outside the home, and Jerome and Jason stay with a neighbor after school for 2 hours each day until their parents return home from work. Mr. and Mrs. Jones are very devoted to the children and are involved in their activities. Jerome and Jason were healthy children, experiencing only an occasional upper respiratory infection, until 4 years ago when Jerome was diagnosed with acute myelocytic leukemia and was treated with chemotherapy. He achieved remission and remained symptom free for 2 years, at which time he experienced relapse and has been undergoing chemotherapy without achieving remission since.

Case Study   The health care providers discuss Jerome's condition with him and with his family, suggesting that Jerome receive a bone marrow transplantation (BMT). After discussing the procedure and potential risks of BMT, Jerome's parents decide to begin the process of finding a suitable donor. They are very anxious about the procedure but understand that without the BMT, Jerome's prognosis is poor. Once a suitable donor is located, Jerome will be admitted to a research hospital that specializes in transplantation in children. The facility is located a 45-minute driving distance from the Jones' home in a neighboring city.

Questions

1. What types of conditions are treated with BMT?

2. Discuss the different types of bone marrow transplants.

3. Jerome's parents ask the nurse about the difference between bone marrow and stem cells. What is the most appropriate explanation for the nurse to give?

4. Discuss the difference between Jerome's assent for the BMT and his parents' informed consent.

5. Why is it important for Jerome to be involved in the decision about whether he should have a BMT and to give his assent?

6. After testing his family, Jason is determined to be a compatible donor. What process determines a compatible donor?

7. Discuss the harvesting and processing of donor bone marrow.

8. Discuss the adverse effects of high-dose chemotherapy and radiation administered prior to BMT.

9. Jerome receives his bone marrow transplant. What are the nursing priorities for his care after his BMT?

10. What is engraftment and how long does it take following a BMT?

11. Discuss the short-term and long-term complications of BMT.

12. Discuss the potential impact of the BMT on Jerome's growth and development.

13. Three months after his BMT, Jerome develops erythema of the palms of his hands, the soles of his feet, and his ears. Discuss your impressions of Jerome's manifestations.

14. Differentiate acute graft-versus-host disease (GVHD) and chronic GVHD.

15. Discuss the techniques used to prevent GVHD.

16. Following treatment, Jerome's parents are preparing to take him home. Discuss appropriate client/family teaching needed prior to Jerome's discharge.

Chad

GENDER	**SOCIOECONOMIC**
M	■ Middle class
AGE	**SPIRITUAL**
10	■ Strength from spirituality
SETTING	**PHARMACOLOGIC**
■ Home	■ Highly active antiretroviral therapy
ETHNICITY	**PSYCHOSOCIAL**
■ White American	■ Death of mother 6 years ago
CULTURAL CONSIDERATIONS	■ Client anxiety
	■ Family anxiety
PREEXISTING CONDITIONS	**LEGAL**
■ HIV	
COEXISTING CONDITIONS	**ETHICAL**
SIGNIFICANT HISTORY	**ALTERNATIVE THERAPY**
COMMUNICATION	**PRIORITIZATION**
	■ Yes
DISABILITY	**DELEGATION**
	■ Yes

THE LYMPHATIC SYSTEM

Level of difficulty: Difficult

Overview: This case requires knowledge of HIV/AIDS, growth and development, grief and grieving, as well as an understanding of the client's background, personal situation, and family relationship.

DIFFICULT

Client Profile

Chad is a 10-year-old boy who contracted human immunodeficiency virus (HIV) from his mother while she was pregnant with him. She had contracted HIV from a blood transfusion following the birth of Chad's older brother, Steve, when she developed disseminated intravascular coagulation (DIC). His mother died when Chad was 4 years old of complications of acquired immunodeficiency syndrome (AIDS). Chad, his father, and brother were tested for HIV following his mother's diagnosis. His father and brother were HIV negative, but Chad was HIV positive. Chad's father remarried when Chad was 6 years old and Chad's stepmother has been very attentive to Chad during his illness. She recently quit work to stay at home with him as his condition worsened. Chad and his family have a large support network including grandparents, aunts, uncles, cousins, and classmates of both Chad and Steve.

Case Study

During a home health visit the nurse notes that Chad has developed skin lesions, a dry cough, and the presence of crackles on auscultation of his breath sounds. His vital signs are:

> Temperature: 38.8° C (101.8° F)
>
> Pulse: 116 beats/minute
>
> Respirations: 28 breaths/minute
>
> Blood pressure: 130/84

She also notes white patches in his mouth. His stepmother says that he has had diarrhea for the past month that he just told her about this morning. She had noticed an increase in his fluid intake, but he told her that he was "just more thirsty" than usual. The nurse notifies the health care provider of her findings, whereupon the physician prescribes a complete blood count and a CDT4 level. Those results are:

> CDT4: 186/mm³, which has decreased from his previous count of 300/mm³
>
> Hemoglobin: 7.8 g/dL
>
> Hematocrit: 20%
>
> Leukocyte count: 1,200/mm³ with a neutrophil count of 900/mm³
>
> Platelet count: 90,000/mm³

Chad weighs 25 kg (55 lb). He had lost 10 pounds in the last month.

Questions

1. Discuss your impressions of the client's assessment data.

2. What additional information would support your impressions?

3. Discuss the significance of Chad's CDT4 count.

4. What are the nursing priorities of care for Chad?

5. Discuss the appropriate priority nursing interventions for Chad.

6. Discuss highly active antiretroviral therapy (HAART) and the classifications and examples of agents used in this treatment regimen.

7. Discuss the medications used to treat common opportunistic infections.

8. The home health nurse notes that Chad is withdrawn today during her visit. His parents confirm that he has not interacted with them "much" for the past week and when he does "he bites our heads off." How would you respond to his parents to help them understand Chad's reaction?

9. Discuss Chad's level of growth and development and how his condition may impact this.

10. Chad says to the home health nurse that he doesn't want his parents to know that his condition is worse because he doesn't want them to worry and he doesn't want to go back to the hospital. What are your impressions of Chad's remarks?

11. On one of the home health nurse's visits, Chad tells the nurse that he misses going to church with his family on Sundays and asks the nurse to pray with him. Discuss Chad's requests and how the nurse might best respond to Chad.

CASE STUDY 4

Ashlee

GENDER	**SOCIOECONOMIC**
F	
AGE	**SPIRITUAL**
4	■ Spiritual strength
SETTING	**PHARMACOLOGIC**
■ Hospital	■ Acetaminophen (Tylenol)
ETHNICITY	■ Ondansetron (Zofran)
■ White American	■ Dexamethasone (Hexadrol)
CULTURAL CONSIDERATIONS	■ Lorazepam (Ativan)
	PSYCHOSOCIAL
PREEXISTING CONDITIONS	■ Local extended family
	■ Client anxiety
	■ Parent anxiety
COEXISTING CONDITIONS	**LEGAL**
SIGNIFICANT HISTORY	**ETHICAL**
COMMUNICATION	**ALTERNATIVE THERAPY**
DISABILITY	**PRIORITIZATION**
	■ Yes
	DELEGATION

THE LYMPHATIC SYSTEM

Level of difficulty: Difficult

Overview: This case requires knowledge of leukemia, growth and development, hospitalization of a preschooler and its impact on the family, as well as an understanding of the client's background and family–child relationship.

DIFFICULT

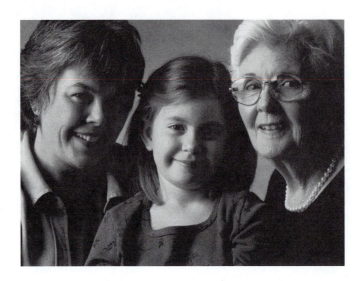

Client Profile

Ashlee is a 4-year-old preschooler who lives with her parents and two older siblings in a suburban environment. She attends preschool five mornings a week and enjoys playing with her 5-year-old sister and 7-year-old brother. She is very active and enjoys playing outside, riding her tricycle, climbing on the family's jungle gym, and playing on the swing set. Her vocabulary consists of approximately 1,500 words and she speaks using four- or five-word sentences. Her parents are very attentive to their children and spend each weekend doing "family activities." During the week, her parents work, and Ashlee and her siblings stay with their grandmother after school. Their grandmother lives in the same neighborhood. In the evenings, the family eats together and maintains an evening schedule that allows for family play time.

Case Study

During the past 2 months, Ashlee has been less active than usual and has begun taking one or two naps in the afternoon. Her grandmother and parents think she looks pale, reasoning that it is because of her high activity level, until her interest in going outside to play decreases dramatically. When they take her temperature, it is elevated so they administer acetaminophen without effect. At this point they decide to take her to see her pediatrician. Although the health care provider found Ashlee's manifestations consistent with an upper respiratory infection, Dr. Polster is concerned and decides to admit Ashlee to the hospital for tests to rule out leukemia.

Questions

1. What diagnostic tests would you expect to be prescribed for Ashlee?

2. Her admission vital signs are:

Temperature: 38° C (100.4° F)
Pulse: 120 beats/minute

Respirations: 28 breaths/minute
Blood pressure: 100/60
and her admission complete blood count reveals:

Hemoglobin: 11 g/dL
Hematocrit: 31%

Erythrocyte count: 4.6 million/mm³

Platelet count: 130,000/mm³

White blood cell count: 4,000 cells/mm³

Neutrophils: 1,600 cells/mm³

Lymphocytes: 1,200 cells/mm³

Monocytes: 290 cells/mm³

Eosinophils: 120 cells/mm³

Basophils: 30 cells/mm³

Discuss the significance of Ashlee's vital signs and laboratory findings.

3. The tests confirm a diagnosis of acute lymphocytic leukemia. Compare the two most common types of childhood leukemia.

4. Ashlee's mother is at Ashlee's bedside crying. As you approach her, she says, "How could God let my little girl get leukemia? What can I do to make it go away?" How would you respond to Ashlee's mother?

5. What are the nursing priorities of care for Ashlee?

6. Discuss the appropriate priority nursing interventions for Ashlee.

7. Discuss the factors that affect Ashlee's prognosis.

8. Ashlee's mother expresses concern because Ashlee "has been potty-trained for 2 years, but she has wet the bed since she has been in the hospital." How would you respond to Ashee's mother?

9. Ashlee's chemotherapy regimen is started and the oncologist prescribes that she receive ondansetron 2.5 mg IV prior to chemotherapy and the same dose every 4 hours for 24 hours. In addition, she prescribes dexamethasone 16 mg IV prior to chemotherapy. Finally, lorazepam 1 mg IV q4h PRN for breakthrough nausea. Discuss these prescriptions including drug classifications, when medications should be administered, special considerations when administering drugs, and safe dosage for Ashlee, who weighs 16.7 kg (36.7 lb).

10. Discuss Ashlee's level of growth and development and how her treatment may impact this.

11. How would you work with Ashlee's parents to help prevent complications associated with her growth and development?

Nicole

GENDER	**SOCIOECONOMIC**
F	
AGE	**SPIRITUAL**
13	
SETTING	**PHARMACOLOGIC**
■ Hospital	■ Acetaminophen (Tylenol)
ETHNICITY	■ Cyclophosphomide (Cytoxan)
■ Middle Eastern	■ Gentamicin sulfate (Garamycin)
CULTURAL CONSIDERATIONS	■ Vancomycin hydrochloride (Vancocin)
	■ Cefoxitin sodium (Mefoxin)
PREEXISTING CONDITIONS	**PSYCHOSOCIAL**
■ Leukemia	
■ Alopecia	**LEGAL**
■ CVAD	
COEXISTING CONDITIONS	**ETHICAL**
SIGNIFICANT HISTORY	**ALTERNATIVE THERAPY**
COMMUNICATION	**PRIORITIZATION**
	■ Yes
DISABILITY	**DELEGATION**

DIFFICULT

THE LYMPHATIC SYSTEM

Level of difficulty: Difficult

Overview: This case requires knowledge of chemotherapy, growth and development, as well as an understanding of the client's background, personal situation, and parent–child relationship.

Client Profile

Nicole is a 13-year-old-with leukemia. She lives at home with her parents and younger siblings and for the past 3 months has been receiving chemotherapy. She has a central venous access device (CVAD) that is cared for by her parents and herself. Nicole has experienced a number of absences from school as a result of her hospitalizations, chemotherapy, and the effects of her chemotherapy regimen, although she has had a tutor at home to keep her current with her studies. Nicole has alopecia and has been hospitalized with a line infection, stomatitis and esophagitis, and bleeding requiring platelet replacement. She refuses to see her friends although she speaks with them frequently on the phone. She tells them her refusal is based on the fact that she is prone to infection and doesn't want to risk exposure and have to be hospitalized again.

Case Study

Nicole is admitted to the pediatric unit of the local hospital with a temperature of 38.8° C (101.8° F) that did not respond to the acetaminophen that she has been taking every 4 hours since yesterday. Her admission assessment indicated that Nicole's lung sounds are clear, heart sounds are strong and regular, she is in no apparent distress, has alopecia, and has evidence of white patches in her mouth. Her laboratory values include:

Hematology:

Hemoglobin: 10.1 g/dL

Hematocrit: 25%

Platelets: 50,000/mm³

White blood cell count: 2,000/mm³

Differential: Neutrophils 20%

Questions

1. Discuss the significance of Nicole's laboratory findings.

2. What other assessment data would be helpful for the nurse to have to prepare Nicole's care plan?

3. What are the priorities of care for Nicole on admission?

4. Discuss the common complications (adverse effects) of chemotherapy.

5. What nursing actions address the adverse effects associated with chemotherapy?

6. Nicole is receiving cyclophosphamide intravenously. Discuss this agent including any nursing interventions necessary specifically related to its use.

7. Nicole is diagnosed with a CVAD line infection. Discuss how these infections occur and why.

8. Nicole's mother is staying with Nicole during her hospitalization and expresses concern about Nicole refusing to see her friends and that Nicole seems "down" since her last chemotherapy. Discuss your impressions about Nicole's mother's statements, considering Nicole's level of growth and development.

9. Nicole tells the nurse that her mouth and throat are so sore she cannot drink or eat anything. Discuss your impressions about Nicole's complaints and the appropriate nursing actions to help Nicole.

10. Nicole is prescribed intravenous antibiotic therapy to treat her line infection. The health care provider prescribes gentamicin sulfate 100 mg IV q8h, vancomycin hydrochloride 500 mg IV every

6 hours, and cefoxitin sodium 1 g IV every 6 hours. Nicole weighs 40 kg (88 lb). Discuss these agents and if the doses prescribed are safe for Nicole.

11. The pharmacy schedules Nicole's antibiotic therapy as follows:

Gentamicin 2400h 0600h 1200h 1800h

Vancomycin 0200h 0800h 1400h 2200h

Cefoxitin 2400h 0600h 1200h 1800h

Discuss this schedule and what alterations the nurse should make, if any.

12. Calculate the rates of administration via a volumetric intravenous infusion pump for the following:

Gentamicin sulfate: 100 mg in 100 mL of 5% dextrose in water to infuse over 30 minutes

Vancomycin hydrochloride: 500 mg in 250 mL of 0.9% normal saline

Cefoxitin sodium :1 g in 50 mL of 5% dextrose in water to infuse over 15 minutes

Katie

GENDER	**SOCIOECONOMIC**
F	
AGE	**SPIRITUAL**
11	
SETTING	**PHARMACOLOGIC**
■ Health care provider's office	■ Acetaminophen (Tylenol)
ETHNICITY	■ Nystatin (Mycostatin)
	■ Prednisone (deltasone)
■ Black American	■ Ibuprofen (Motrin)
CULTURAL CONSIDERATIONS	**PSYCHOSOCIAL**
	■ Client anxiety
PREEXISTING CONDITIONS	**LEGAL**
COEXISTING CONDITIONS	**ETHICAL**
SIGNIFICANT HISTORY	**ALTERNATIVE THERAPY**
COMMUNICATION	**PRIORITIZATION**
	■ Yes
DISABILITY	**DELEGATION**
	■ Client teaching

THE LYMPHATIC SYSTEM

Level of difficulty: Difficult

Overview: This case requires knowledge of systemic lupus erythematosus (SLE), growth and development, as well as an understanding of the client's background, personal situation, and parent–child relationship, and of interaction with antagonistic parents.

DIFFICULT

Client Profile

Katie is an 11-year-old schoolage child who lives with her parents and 13-year-old sister in a suburban neighborhood. She has a 2-year history of frequent upper respiratory infections (URI) accompanied by joint pain, headaches, and mouth ulcers. Her parents are frustrated because even though Katie's pediatrician has treated her recurrent URIs, no definitive diagnosis has been made to explain her other clinical manifestations. They treat her headaches and joint pain with acetaminophen and the mouth ulcers with nystatin, but they continue to recur. Her symptoms have caused Katie's school performance to decline, and now over the past 2 days, Katie has developed a malar rash in the shape of a butterfly. Determined to find out what is wrong with Katie, her parents make another appointment to see her pediatrician.

Case Study

Katie is brought to her pediatrician's office by her parents. As the nurse approaches them, Katie's mother says, "We haven't seen you here before but either you people find out what is wrong with Katie and effectively treat her or we are going to find another pediatrician who knows what he is doing." During her assessment, the nurse notes that Katie is pale and holding her head in her hand. When questioned, Katie says, "Oh, it's just another one of my headaches. I probably have a brain tumor like my friend Alisha." Katie's vital signs are: temperature, 37.7° C; pulse, 115 beats/minute; respirations, 24 breaths/minute; and blood pressure, 112/70.

Questions

1. Discuss your impression of Katie's history and clinical manifestations.

2. What other assessment data would be helpful for the nurse to have to prepare Katie's care plan?

3. Discuss her parents' comment to the nurse and how the nurse can best respond to them.

4. Discuss Katie's comment and how the nurse can best respond to her.

5. Katie is diagnosed with SLE. What is SLE and why is it so difficult to diagnose?

6. How common is SLE in children?

7. Discuss the potential complications associated with SLE.

8. What are the priorities of care for Katie during this visit?

9. Discuss the impact of Katie's clinical manifestations and diagnosis on her growth and development.

10. Katie is prescribed prednisone 5 mg by mouth each day, ibuprofen 200 mg by mouth every 6 hours as needed for pain, and acetaminophen 320 mg by mouth every 4–6 hours (alternating with ibuprofen) as needed for pain. Katie weighs 78.1 lb. Discuss these prescriptions including drug classifications, use in treating SLE, and whether the prescribed doses are safe for Katie.

11. Discuss the pre-discharge teaching priorities for Katie and her parents.

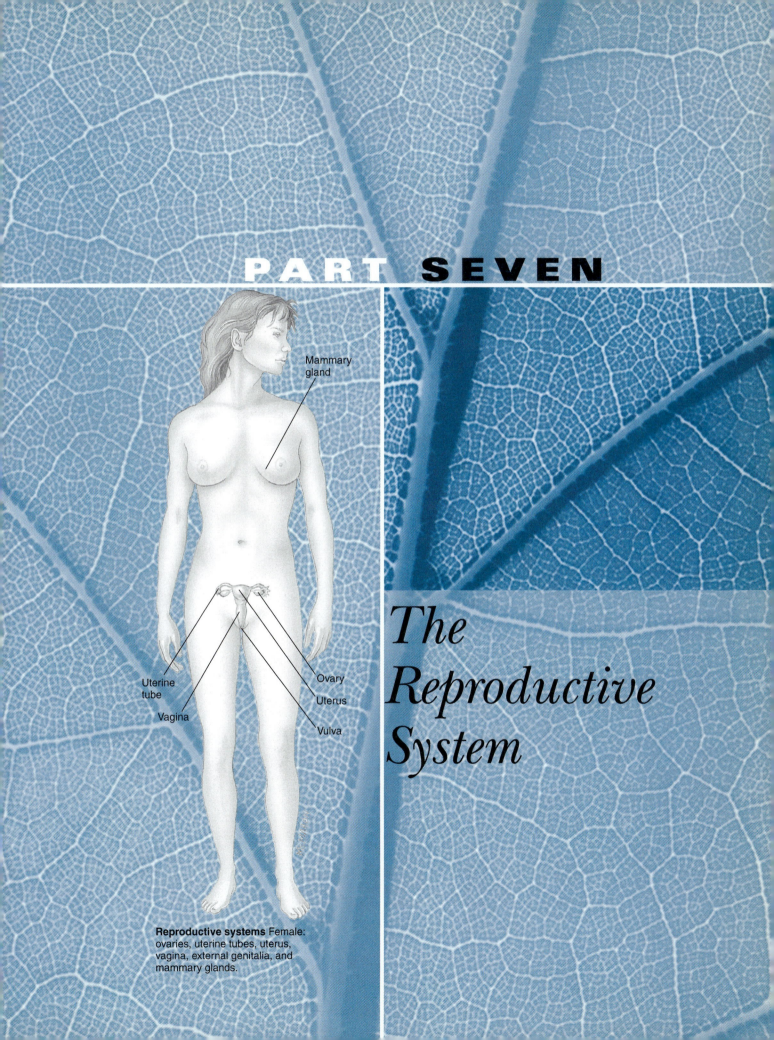

PART SEVEN

The Reproductive System

Mammary gland

Uterine tube

Vagina

Ovary

Uterus

Vulva

Reproductive systems Female: ovaries, uterine tubes, uterus, vagina, external genitalia, and mammary glands.

Sriah

GENDER

F

AGE

3 weeks old

SETTING

■ Home

ETHNICITY

CULTURAL CONSIDERATIONS

■ Iraqi

PREEXISTING CONDITIONS

COEXISTING CONDITIONS

SIGNIFICANT HISTORY

COMMUNICATION

DISABILITY

SOCIOECONOMIC

■ Middle class

SPIRITUAL

■ Muslim

PHARMACOLOGIC

PSYCHOSOCIAL

■ Breastfeeding support

LEGAL

ETHICAL

ALTERNATIVE THERAPY

PRIORITIZATION

DELEGATION

THE REPRODUCTIVE SYSTEM

Level of difficulty: Easy

Overview: This case requires knowledge of breastfeeding and alternative options as well as understanding of the client's culture, background, personal situation, and mother–child attachment relationship.

Client Profile

Sriah is a 3-week-old infant who was born at 37 weeks' gestation following premature labor. She weighed 2.3 kg (5 lb, 1 oz) at birth. Her mother immigrated to the United States from Iraq 8 months ago shortly after becoming pregnant. She had studied English in her home country before immigrating. In the United States she attended prenatal classes with her husband, followed her prescribed nutritional program, and during her prenatal classes decided to breastfeed her baby. Sriah is nursing every 2–3 hours for 20 minutes each feeding and has eight wet diapers a day. Because of her low birth weight, she is seen at her pediatrician's office, at which time she weighs 2.6 kg (5 lb, 11 oz). She receives weekly visits from the home health nurse to monitor Sriah's growth progress.

Case Study

Sriah's mother tells the home health nurse that her mother-in-law came to visit during her seventh month of pregnancy and remains with them to "help with the baby." She states that her mother-in-law is very concerned that Sriah is not getting enough nutrition with the breastfeeding and repeatedly tells her son and daughter that Sriah should be on formula. Sriah is frequently fussy after eating, and her grandmother states that the breastfeeding is responsible for Sriah's discomfort and Sriah's father is not supportive about the breastfeeding, agreeing with his mother. As a result, Sriah's mother is considering stopping the breastfeeding and starting formula feeding because "it would probably be better for Sriah."

Questions

1. Discuss your impressions about the above situation.

2. Discuss the normal weight gain for an infant Sriah's age and compare it to Sriah's current weight.

3. Discuss the advantages of breastfeeding, including those specific to Sriah's situation.

4. What factors indicate that Sriah is receiving adequate nutrition from her mother's breastfeeding?

5. Discuss the possible relationship between Sriah's discomfort following feedings and breastfeeding in this family situation.

6. Given the dietary intake consistent with Sriah's family's culture, what, if any, relationship might this have on Sriah's discomfort following feedings?

7. Discuss the significance of family support when a mother wants to breastfeed her infant.

8. Identify the priority nursing diagnoses pertinent to this situation.

9. Discuss how the nurse could intervene in this situation to support the mother's desire to breastfeed Sriah.

10. During the visit, Sriah's mother decides to continue breastfeeding with her husband and mother-in-law's support. What, if any, professionals should the nurse collaborate with regarding this situation to ensure adequate and consistent follow-up for Sriah and her family?

Alexis

GENDER	**SOCIOECONOMIC STATUS**
F	
AGE	**SPIRITUAL**
16	
SETTING	**PHARMACOLOGIC**
■ Prenatal clinic	
ETHNICITY	**PSYCHOSOCIAL**
■ White American	■ Single pregnant teenager
CULTURAL CONSIDERATIONS	**LEGAL**
PREEXISTING CONDITIONS	**ETHICAL**
■ Pregnant	■ Possible nurse bias
COEXISTING CONDITIONS	**ALTERNATIVE THERAPY**
SIGNIFICANT HISTORY	**PRIORITIZATION**
COMMUNICATION	**DELEGATION**
	■ Yes
DISABILITY	

MODERATE

THE REPRODUCTIVE SYSTEM

Level of difficulty: Moderate

Overview: This case requires knowledge of growth and development, pregnancy, parenting, prenatal mental health, as well as an understanding of the client's personal situation and family relationships.

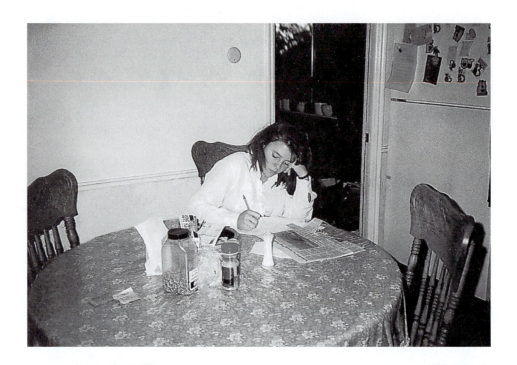

Client Profile

Alexis is a 16-year-old high school sophomore who is single and living at home with her parents. Her boyfriend Matt, who is the father of the child she is carrying, is an 18-year-old senior at the same high school Alexis attends. Alexis and Matt, who also lives at home with his parents a few houses away from Alexis and her parents, have been going together since he was a sophomore and she was in eighth grade. They both have excelled in school and were very popular with their classmates until the last semester, at which time their grades began to falter and their popularity diminished. They appear to care a great deal for each other, but both had plans to attend college after high school graduation, and in the past month they have argued frequently. Both Matt and Alexis' parents have been very supportive, although initially they were devastated by the news of the pregnancy.

Case Study

During her prenatal visit during her 32nd week of her first pregnancy, Alexis states she has been experiencing low back pain and "tightening in my tummy" for the past week. When a vaginal examination is performed, it reveals that her cervix is 0 cm dilated, thick, and high with no evidence of effacement. Alexis appears irritable, stating, "I just want this to be over. I'm tired of being big and fat while my friends are pretty and doing all the things I want to be doing. Can't you just take the baby now? A friend of mine had her baby early and she and the baby are just fine." Alexis is accompanied by her parents and Matt, who have attended all of her prenatal visits with her.

Questions

1. Discuss your impressions about the above situation.

2. What additional data would be helpful in developing a plan of care for Alexis?

3. How do Alexis' growth and development needs differ from those of a 28-year-old woman?

4. Given their psychosocial level of growth and development, discuss how you think Alexis and Matt are feeling about their situation.

5. How would you respond to Alexis' statement about premature births?

6. How effective do you think your teaching about premature births would be to Alexis at this time?

7. Discuss your impressions of Alexis and Matt's parents' response to the pregnancy.

8. Discuss your biases, if any, toward Alexis' situation.

9. What impact would your biases, if any, have on your approach to Alexis and Matt?

10. Discuss your teaching plan for Alexis and her significant others at this visit.

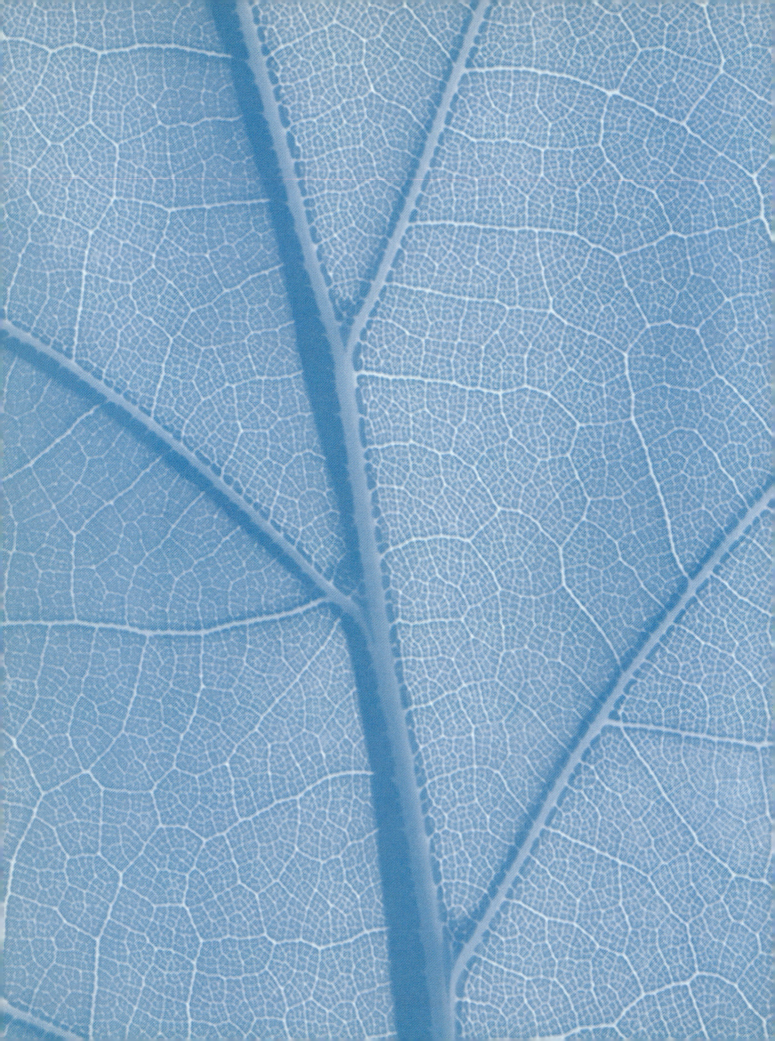

Index

Index